Workbook to Accompany

Essentials of Immunology & Serology

Jacqueline Stanley, Ph.D.

St. George's University School of Medicine
St. George's, Grenada, West Indies

Written by

F. Christopher Sowers, M.S.

Wilkes Community College
Wilkesboro, North Carolina

THOMSON

DELMAR LEARNING

Australia Canada Mexico Singapore Spain United Kingdom United States

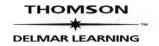

THOMSON

DELMAR LEARNING

Workbook to Accompany
Essentials of Immunology & Serology
Jacqueline Stanley
written by F. Christopher Sowers

Health Care Publishing Director: William Brottmiller
Executive Editor: Cathy L. Experti
Acquisitions Editor: Maureen Rosener
Developmental Editor: Darcy M. Scelsi

Editorial Assistant: Matthew Thouin
Executive Marketing Manager: Dawn F. Gerrain
Channel Manager: Jennifer McAvey
Production Editor: James Zayicek

For permission to use material from this text or product, contact us by
Tel   (800) 730-2214
Fax   (800) 730-2215

ISBN 0-7668-1065-8

NOTICE TO THE READER

The Publisher and the authors do not warrant or guarantee any of the products described herein or perform any independent analysis in connection with any of the product information contained herein. The publisher and the authors do not assume and expressly disclaim any obligation to obtain and include information other than that provided by the manufacturer.

The reader is expressly warned to consider and adopt all safety precautions that might be indicated by the activities described herein and to avoid all potential hazards. By following the instructions contained herein, the reader willingly assumes all risks in connection with such instructions.

The publisher and the authors make no representations or warranties of any kind, including but not limited to the warranties of fitness for a particular purpose or merchantability nor are any such representations implied with respect to the material set forth herein, and the publisher and the authors take no responsibility with respect to such material. The publisher and the authors shall not be liable for any special, consequential, or exemplary damages resulting, in whole or in part, from the reader's use of, or reliance upon, this material.

The authors and publisher have made a conscientious effort to ensure that the drug information and recommended dosages in this book are accurate and in accord with accepted standards at the time of publication. However, pharmacology and therapeutics are rapidly changing sciences, so readers are advised, before administering any drug, to check the package insert provided by the manufacturer for the recommended dose, for any contraindications for administration, and for any added warnings and precautions. This recommendation is especially important for new, infrequently used, or highly toxic drugs.

CONTENTS

PREFACE

This workbook is a companion to *Essentials of Immunology & Serology*. It is designed to help reinforce the concepts presented in each chapter of the text and to help in the application of these concepts.

The exercises in the workbook were developed from the content in the core text. For effective study completing a chapter in the text is recommended prior to beginning the related chapter in the workbook.

Each chapter begins with the learning objectives from the text. This repetition is intended to help focus on the important goals established for each chapter. Read through each objective to see how many you are able to meet. Keep track of those that you are unable to answer so you can return to that section for further study.

A variety of review questions are also provided based upon each chapter content. Types of questions include multiple choice, matching, true false, and completion. There are also critical thinking questions to help you hone your ability to problem solve. Answers to the questions appear at the end of the book.

Section I

FUNCTIONS OF THE IMMUNE SYSTEM AND IMMUNITY

CHAPTER 1

AN OVERVIEW OF THE IMMUNE SYSTEM

OUTLINE

- Historical Perspective
- An Introduction to the Immune System
  - Innate Immunity
  - Adaptive Immunity
- Overview of Innate and Adaptive Immune Integration
  - Custom Made Assault
- Immunodeficiencies
  - Secondary Immunodeficiency Disorders

OBJECTIVES

Upon completion of this chapter, the reader should be able to:

1. Discuss in general terms the immune system from a historical perspective.
2. Discuss the general characteristics of innate immunity.
3. List the various mechanisms classed as innate immunity and discuss their role in host defense.
4. List the various mechanisms classed as adaptive immunity and discuss their role in host defense.
5. Compare the basic features of innate and adaptive immunity.
6. Identify the cells that play a role in innate immunity and adaptive immunity.

7. Provide a general description of the role of innate and adaptive immune systems in response to organisms as a function of their location in the body.

8. Discuss various conditions that result in immunosuppression.

SUMMARY OF KEY POINTS

Immunology is characterized by (i) discrimination between self and non-self, and (ii) elimination of non-self. Non-self can be defined as any component such as infectious agents or pathogens the body recognizes, and then works to remove. Soluble molecules, many different types of cells, and tissues throughout the body make up the immune system. The immune system is therefore complex with many components and these factors interact with one another producing activation, regulation, or inhibition of the immune response. These responses are usually considered as either innate or adaptive for academic reasons, and in reality both innate and adaptive immunity work together synchronously, and both can be seen as humoral and cellular.

Innate immunity is not specific to any one foreign protein or antigen, nor does it possess a cellular memory. Anatomical barriers like the skin, cilia, and mucus; resident flora like non pathogenic bacteria (e.g., *Staphylococcus epidermis*); cells like phagocytes, antigen presenting cells, and natural killer cells; and humoral factors like lysozyme, pepsin, or lactoferrin all represent host defenses in innate immunity.

Adaptive immunity adapts to specific antigens. Lymphocytes, activated in adaptive immunity, have cell surface receptors specific for an antigen, and once lymphocytes interact with a particular antigen, they will respond much faster to subsequent exposure. This is cellular memory, and along with specificity to an antigen, it is characteristic of adaptive immunity. Cell types like B cells and T helper cells, and humoral factors like antibodies and cytokines represent host defenses in adaptive immunity.

When some essential part of the immune system is lacking or not working properly then immunodeficiency disorders occur. Immunodeficiencies can be primary and genetic, or secondary and lifestyle related. Whether primary or secondary, these immunodeficiencies demonstrate how effective the immune system is in maintaining our health normally.

Many genetic defects are known in almost all parts of the immune system, which result in primary immunodeficiency. Secondary immunosuppression is usually associated with a decrease in helper T cells and the cytokines they secrete, and viral infections, post transplant and cancer therapies, malnutrition, diabetes, alcohol, stress, and aging are all examples of secondary immunodeficiency.

REVIEW OF KEY TERMS AND ABBREVIATIONS

Matching: Match the key term in the left column with the definition in the right column.

1. _K_ adaptive immunity

a) APCs, basophils, eosinophils, mast cells, phagocytes

2. _t_ anatomical barriers

b) worms

3. _G_ antigen

c) when activated, some will differentiate into plasma cells

4. _O_ antigen presenting cells

d) cleaves the cell wall of a class of bacteria

5. _Q_ apoptosis

6. _C_ B cells

7. _M_ basophils

8. _A_ cellular factors

9. _N_ cilia

10. _H_ clonal expansion

11. _P_ complement system

12. _E_ cytokines

13. _J_ eosinophils

14. _B_ helminths

15. _f_ helper T cell

16. _L_ humoral factors

17. _R_ immunological memory

18. _U_ innate immunity

19. _I_ lactoferrin

20. _D_ lysozyme

21. _S_ pathogens

e) communication proteins secreted by immune cells

f) secrete humoral factors called cytokines

g) foreign substances that cause an immune response

h) lymphocytes divide until there is a large colony of cells

i) binds iron restricting amount available to bacteria

j) important role in destruction of helminths

k) characteristics are specificity and memory

l) substances, usually proteins, present in bodily fluids

m) facilitate recruitment of immune cells to infection site

n) in respiratory tract; force particles upward

o) adaptive immune responses cannot occur without these

p) more than 30 proteins; destroy extracellular bacteria

q) "cell suicide"

r) more efficient response upon subsequent infection

s) microorganisms that can cause disease

t) consist primarily of skin, mucous membranes, and cilia

u) characterized by no memory and no specificity

Definitions: Write the definition of each of the following words or terms.

1. membrane antibodies   _____

_____

2. membrane immunoglobulins   _____

_____

3. mucous membranes   _____

_____

4. natural killer cells   _____

_____

5. mast cells   _____

_____

6. pepsin   _____

_____

7. phagocytes   _____

_____

8. plasma cells   _____

_____

9. recognition   _____

_____

10. resident flora   _____

_____

11. skin   _____

_____

12. stomach acidity   _____

_____

13. T cells _____

_____

REVIEW EXERCISES

True or False: Read each statement and decide if it is TRUE or FALSE. Place T or F on the line before each statement.

1. _F_   The immune system functions pretty much autonomously.

2. _F_   A characteristic of innate immunity is humoral specificity.

3. _T_   Immune responses depend on the type of infection.

4. _F_   Primary immunodeficiencies are acquired by lifestyle.

5. _T_   Humoral immunity deals with substances in body fluids.

Fill in the Blank: Complete the following sentences on the immune system by filling in the missing word or words.

1. The immune system's ability to distinguish between self and non-self is _recognition_

2. _resident flora_ are nonpathogenic bacteria in the intestine, vagina, and nasopharynx.

3. B cells that secrete antibodies are called _plasma cells_

4. Cells that eliminate other cells infected with viruses are called _cytotoxic T. killer cell_

5. _Helper T cells_ are cells that secrete soluble proteins called cytokines.

Multiple Choice: Choose the best answer.

1. What is the protection arising from an exposure to an antigen (like the ancient Chinese custom of inhaling powder from the crusts of lesions from individuals recovering from small pox) called?

    a. immunology
    b. infection
    c. recognition
    d. vaccination
    e. anatomical barrier

2. Whether a component of the immune system is classified innate or adaptive depends on what two criteria?

    a. specificity and antigens
    b. specificity and presence of resident flora
    c. killer cells and anatomical barriers
    d. resolution of infection and memory
    e. specificity and memory

3. What anatomical defense mechanism forces particles upward where they can be either swallowed or eliminated during the cough reflex?

   a. cilia
   b. mucous membranes
   c. skin
   d. mucus
   e. resident flora

4. Humoral defense mechanisms would include which of the following?

   a. phagocytes
   b. lysozyme
   c. natural killer cells
   d. basophils
   e. plasma cells

5. When would you expect apoptosis (cell suicide) to occur?

   a. with clonal expansion
   b. recognition and interaction
   c. after elimination of antigen or infectious agent
   d. immunosurveillance of memory cells
   e. activation of innate and adaptive immunity

CRITICAL THINKING EXERCISES

Critical Thinking 1: Read this scenario and then answer the questions that follow.

Tom from immunology comes up to you after class one day and says: "I don't know what the big deal is anyway. Whether you say acquired or adapted, they both mean responses that are specific and have a cellular memory, and an immediate response is just that, and nothing more. I mean, after all, immunity is the specificity really, isn't it? Why not talk about general resistance instead of innate immunity, like a lot of other books?"

1. What could you tell Tom to convince him that the term "adapted" really does make more sense? Where did Tom get the term "acquired" anyway?

2. How would you explain to Tom why it is better to think of innate and adapted processes both together as immunity, instead of two separate processes?

3. Is Tom looking at this from a historical research perspective? What identifies that viewpoint in his statements? What can you let Tom in on that may change his mind?

Critical Thinking 2: Read this scenario and then answer the questions that follow.

Sarah from your immunology class was paraphrasing from the chapter on immunity when she said: "Awareness of exposure to something infectious resulting in protection upon re-exposure to that same infectious agent was the birth of immunology." You replied to Sarah's statement by saying: "Ah yes, but the essence of immunology is the discrimination between self and non-self."

1. What immune factor essentially integrates the immune system functioning, and finally, the resolution (or not) of infection? Does this help explain recognition? Why or why not?

2. How do you reconcile the random arrangement of genes resulting in the specific expression of antigen recognizing receptors on lymphocyte cell surfaces? Does this explain recognition? Why or why not?

3. What part do antigen presenting cells play in recognition? Does this explain recognition? Why or why not?

Critical Thinking 3: Read this scenario and then answer the questions that follow.

Your study group is reviewing for the exam on the immune system and you are discussing activation, regulation, and inhibition. But Sarah is still thinking about recognition, and she says: "I really cannot get past a list of components for the immune system. The chapter is filled with lists, so I suppose it is all that is really important. Besides, my head hurts with all this complexity." Tom, still wanting to see two different processes working separately, chimes in with: "That's right. If they didn't want us to think about two things and their separate parts, the chapter would have been written differently. And, then what about this humoral and cellular difference for both?"

1. How might you take charge of this study session "mutiny" and patiently explain what they obviously didn't read carefully enough? What is getting them off the mark?

2. How do immune system interactions and little autonomous function help pull all the seemingly separate immune system facts together into a challenging, but unified whole?

3. Why do you suppose Tom is having trouble with humoral and cellular components for both innate and adaptive immunity? What can you say to help him understand, and tie it in with what you had been studying earlier about cells and soluble factors interacting?

CASE STUDY

A 25-year-old clinician has been ill for the last several days, but is better now though still a little weak. Talking with friends after work, the clinician mentions the effects of the illness, which were temperature, headache, general body aches, diarrhea, vomiting, congestion, and coughing. When queried about the cause of the illness, the clinician responds that it was "just a virus," and that he gets it about every other year or so.

1. What is your response to "just a virus?" Discuss pathogens and antigens.

2. From the list of signs and symptoms for this illness, what can you say about what sorts of tissues would be involved in an immune response? What sorts of cells? What sorts of substances (proteins)?

3. Describe innate and adaptive immune responses for this individual. Is it possible to predict whether this clinician will ever have this "virus" again? Why or why not? What processes are involved in the immunity to this "virus?"

CHAPTER 2

ANTIGENS AND ANTIGEN RECOGNITION

OUTLINE

- Antigens
    - Prerequisites for Immunogenicity
    - Relative Immunogenicity of Different Types of Molecules
    - Molecules That Enhance Immunogenicity
- Activators of Lymphocytes
    - Antigens
    - Superantigens
    - Mitogens
- Antigen Recognition
    - Antigen Recognition by Cells of Innate Immunity
    - Antigen Recognition by Cells of Adaptive Immunity

OBJECTIVES

Upon completion of this chapter, the reader should be able to:

1. Describe the characteristics of antigens.
2. Describe the types of biological molecules that are immunogenic, weakly immunogenic, or non-immunogenic.
3. Explain the terms monoclonal activators, oligoclonal activators, and polyclonal activators.
4. Explain the term adjuvant and its role in vaccines.

5. Explain the difference in the way T cells and B cells recognize antigens.
6. Understand how various cells of the innate immune system recognize antigens.

SUMMARY OF KEY POINTS

In this text, the classical definition of antigen referring to substances that induce immune responses is used interchangeably with the newer term immunogen, as are antigenicity and immunogenicity used to refer to the effectiveness of molecules to trigger cells of adaptive immunity. However, antigens bind to antibodies, regardless of whether they necessarily elicit an immune response. Antigen receptors of B cells and T cells only recognize specific regions of the typically large antigen, which are called antigenic determinants or epitopes.

Properties making antigens highly immunogenic are (i) foreignness (e.g., non-self molecules like bacteria), (ii) chemical complexity, and (iii) high molecular weight. In autoimmune diseases, however, the immune system responds to some protein in the body although it is not really foreign, and high molecular weight polysaccharides are not strongly immunogenic since they are relatively homogeneous and not complex. Most potent antigens are of high molecular weight though small molecules called haptens can become immunogenic when coupled with a carrier. Proteins by virtue of their complexity and high molecular weight are the most immunogenic compounds.

Adjuvants are substances that enhance the immune response to an antigen by allowing the antigen to stay in the system for a longer period of time by making it more difficult to destroy and thus available to stimulate appropriate immune cells for a longer period of time. Examples of adjuvants include alum precipitate, MF-59, and Freund's complete adjuvant.

Lymphocytes can be activated by monoclonal activators (antigens), oligoclonal activators (superantigens), and polyclonal activators (mitogens). Antigens are classified as T-dependent (proteins) or T-independent (polysaccharides) based on whether they can activate B cells with or without the presence of T cells. Activation of T cells or B cells following antigen contact creates a population of cells that forms one (mono) clone; superantigens, typically derived from bacteria, activate a subset of T cells, but not all T cells, so a few (oligo) different clones will be present in the population of activated cells; while mitogens are polyclonal activators from typically plant proteins binding to molecules present on virtually all T cells and/or B cells, and many (poly) clones are generated.

Antigen recognition of the cells that function in innate immunity may be direct, with the antigen reacting with a receptor directly or indirectly through another molecule binding the antigen (opsonin). Indirect recognition is especially true for phagocytes, natural killer cells, mast cells, and basophils.

T cells and B cells that are cells functioning in adaptive immunity, recognize antigens differently. B cells recognize epitopes on an intact antigen while T cells recognize epitopes on antigen fragments bound to special proteins. These unique proteins are encoded by a gene complex referred to as the major histocompatibility complex (MHC) and are called MHC molecules or MHC proteins. There are two MHC proteins. Type 1 is recognized by cytotoxic T cells, and type 2 is recognized by helper T cells.

REVIEW OF KEY TERMS AND ABBREVIATIONS

Matching: Match the key term in the left column with the definition in the right column.

1. ___ adjuvant a) effectiveness to trigger adaptive immunity cells

2. ___ tumor specific antigen b) plant protein also known as mitogen

3. _A_ antigenicity

4. _K_ carrier

5. _N_ (B) concanavalin A

6. _E_ Dalton

7. _R_ epitope

8. _S_ hapten

9. _M_ (L) immunogen

10. _F_ T-independent antigens

11. _t_ lipopolysaccharide

12. _l_ MHC

13. _Q_ mitogen

14. _L_ monoclonal activator

15. _H_ oligoclonal activator

16. _C_ opsonin

17. _U_ polyhemagglutinin

18. _J_ pokeweed mitogen

19. _B_ polyclonal activator

20. _D_ recombinant protein

21. _P_ T-dependent antigens

c) antigen bound to another molecule

d) synthetic antigen

e) an atomic mass unit

f) antigens that activate B cells in the absence of T cells

g) substance enhancing immune response to an antigen

h) bacteria-derived; also known as superantigen

i) gene complex acting as potent antigens to someone else

j) a protein that activates both T cells and B cells (PWM)

k) small molecules attach to this to become immunogenic

l) also known as antigen

m) substance capable of producing an immune response

n) a plant glycoprotein that activates T cells

o) protein different from all others in genetic code

p) antigens only activate B cells in the presence of T cells

q) plant protein binds all T & B cells; polyclonal activator

r) specific region of antigen recognized by B & T cells

s) epitope with a carrier; small nonimmunogenic molecule

t) a protein that activates B cells (LPS)

u) a plant glycoprotein that activates T cells

Definitions: Write the definition of each of the following words or terms.

1. tumor specific antigen _____

_____

2. T-dependent antigen _____

_____

3. T-independent antigen _____

_____

4. Con A _____

_____

5. LPS _____

_____

6. MHC _____

_____

7. PHA _____

_____

8. PWM _____

_____

9. hapten _____

_____

10. epitope _____

_____

11. adjuvant _____

_____

12. carrier _____

_____

13. opsonin _____

_____

REVIEW EXERCISES

True or False: Read each statement and decide if it is TRUE or FALSE. Place T or F on the line before each statement.

1. _T_   Antigenic determinants and epitopes are the same thing.

2. _T_   ABO polysaccharides are immunogenic.

3. _F_   Proteins are most immunogenic due to lack of complexity.

4. _T_   In autoimmune disorders nucleic acids are immunogenic.

5. _F_   Adjuvant function is to allow the antigen to be eliminated quickly.

Fill in the Blank: Complete the following sentences on the immune system by filling in the missing word or words.

1. Monoclonal activators are also called _Antigens_ .

2. _Super antigens_ are molecules typically derived from bacteria . (Oligoclonal activators

3. The _Opsinin_ serves as a link between innate cells and the antigen.

4. B cells interact with antigens that are _intact_ .

5. Adaptive cells have receptors that possess _Specificity_

Multiple Choice: Choose the best answer.

1. How do B cells and T cells interact with antigen differently?

   a. B cells interact with antigen fragments.
   b. B cells do not possess specificity.
   c. T cells recognize antigen fragments.
   d. T cells interact with intact antigens.
   e. B and T cells do not react differently with antigen.

2. How might a small molecule become immunogenic?

   a. by binding to a protein carrier as a hapten
   b. because of its high molecular weight
   c. as a T cell receptor
   d. as an opsonin
   e. because they are mitogens

3. What is an example of an adjuvant?

   a. mitogens
   b. concanavalin A
   c. Freund's
   d. superantigens
   e. lipopolysaccharide

4. What molecules are most immunogenic?

   a. polysaccharides
   b. lipids
   c. nucleic acids
   d. proteins
   e. haptens

5. Chemical complexity refers to what characteristic?

   a. high molecular weight of polysaccharides
   b. foreign molecules such as those from pokeweed
   c. molecules greater than one kD, less than 6 kD
   d. many different building blocks, like amino acids, in proteins
   e. alum precipitate, a suspension of aluminum hydroxide mixed with antigen

CRITICAL THINKING EXERCISES

Critical Thinking 1: Read this scenario and then answer the questions that follow.

Some nursing students have been talking to Tom and Sarah from immunology class about their up-coming exam on hematology that includes the ABO blood groups. The nursing students know that certain blood types are not to be mixed in transfusions, but they do not quite understand why this is so. When the nursing students are talking with Tom and Sarah, they mention polysaccharide chains on the outside of RBCs.

1. What do Tom and Sarah tell the nursing students to help them understand?

2. To be completely accurate, and to help them be prepared for their own exam in immunology, what else must Tom and Sarah tell the nursing students about polysaccharides?

3. How much chemistry is necessary for Tom and Sarah to explain all this?

Critical Thinking 2: Read this scenario and then answer the questions that follow.

Tom is reading about opsonins and he is fascinated. He says, "Finally, I have figured out this innate/adaptive recognition thing!" Sarah is not as elated, but she sees that Tom seems to finally be putting the pieces together. He is beginning to understand that innate and adapted processes are both considered immunity by either indirect or direct interaction respectively.

1. What might Sarah ask Tom to see if he really has finally decided to declare a truce and consider both innate and adapted processes as types of immunity?

2. How do opsonins differentiate the innate immune cell from the adaptive immune cell? Is this the essence of recognition, do you think? Why or why not?

3. What does the major histocompatibility complex (MHC) have to do with all of this? And, how do these MHC proteins add another important dimension to recognition?

CASE STUDY

Sarah and Tom have been introduced to a lab technician who is involved with the isolation of monoclonal antibodies. The technician mentions to Tom and Sarah that these molecules are used in diagnostic tests for various diseases like hepatitis and strep throat, as well as detecting cancer. Additionally, Sarah and Tom find out that another lab nearby to this technician's is concerned with work on polyclonal activators.

1. How might Tom and Sarah put the information they read in this chapter on monoclonal activators together with the technician's telling them that he can detect diseases from monoclonal antibodies? What other uses do you think monoclonal antibodies might have?

2. How would monoclonal antibodies be able to detect cancer? Do you think monoclonal antibodies might be able to give you information on the spread of cancer (metastasis)? How useful might that sort of data be to clinicians?

3. What can Tom and Sarah tell the technician about polyclonal activators, and why do you think the lab is interested in polyclonal activators to begin with?

CHAPTER 3

ANTIBODIES

OUTLINE

- Antibodies
  - Gamma Globulins
  - Structure
  - Bifunctional Property of Antibodies
  - Determining Bifunctionality
  - Cross-Reactivity
- Antigen Antibody Interactions
  - Primary Interactions
  - Secondary Interactions
- Classification of Antibodies
  - Isotypes
  - Allotypes
- Properties and Biological Function of Antibody Isotypes
  - Immunoglobulin G
  - Immunoglobulin E
  - Immunoglobulin M
  - Immunoglobulin D
  - Immunoglobulin A
- Quantitation of Serum Antibodies
- Monoclonal Antibodies

OBJECTIVES

Upon completion of this chapter, the reader should be able to:

1. Describe the structure of an antibody molecule and its properties.
2. Classify the various antibody isotypes, their subclasses and variants.
3. Describe the properties and role of the various isotypes.
4. Explain how monoclonal antibodies are generated.
5. Describe the various types of antigen/antibody interactions and the techniques used for measuring these interactions.

SUMMARY OF KEY POINTS

Antibodies (immunoglobulins) are proteins with major roles to play in immune responses that may be on B cell surfaces or a differentiated form of B cell (plasma cells) may secrete them. On the surface of a B cell, the antibodies are referred to as membrane immunoglobulin (mIg), and they have an additional transmembrane sequence permitting insertion and anchorage into the cell membrane; when antibodies are secreted, they are simply referred to as antibodies and do not contain the additional piece. After an antigen activates B cells, then they are differentiated into plasma cells, which secrete the antibodies specific for that antigen.

Electrophoresis, in which proteins are separated under the influence of an electric field, is used to separate secreted antibodies from other serum proteins. Proteins move either toward the positive terminal of the applied electric field (cathode) or toward the negative terminal (anode) based on its net electric charge. Electrophoresis is done by incorporating the serum proteins within a supporting medium (e.g., polyacrylamide) and then exposing them to an electric field in which five distinct bands are isolated from blood serum. The proteins migrating closest to the anode are referred to as gamma globulins, or simply immunoglobulin.

Prototypic monomeric antibody molecules have four polypeptide chains: two that are called light chains and two that are called heavy chains. Each of these chains has a variable region and a constant region, in which the light chain variable regions are made up of "V" and "J" segments, the heavy chain variable regions are made of up "V," "D," and "J" segments. Antibodies bind to antigen via the binding sites made up of the combined variable regions of light and heavy chains. Affinity of an antigen-binding site for a univalent antigen is termed the association constant, whereas a measure of overall binding between antigen-binding sites and multivalent antigen is avidity.

The antigen binding capability and biological functions of an antibody are associated with different regions of the antibody. Antibodies are bifunctional molecules determined from studies showing two different products from two proteolytic enzymes. This demonstrated that one region of the antibody contains the antigen-binding domain, and the other region contained the domain for other biological activities. Some antibodies will show cross-reactivity, binding to an antigenic determinant that is similar, rather than being exactly the same, although antigen-binding sites of antibodies are considered to be very specific; immunization with modified toxins makes use of this property of antibodies.

Classification of antibodies is based on the heavy chain constant region, defining the antibody isotypes: IgM, IgD, IgG, IgE, and IgA. Most antibody isotypes have the constant region genetically the same in all individuals, with minor differences for IgG and IgA in the population. These differences are referred to as allotypes and represent individual differences.

The biological activity of an isotype is in the heavy chain constant region. IgG is the predominant serum antibody with three major roles in host immunity: (1) activation of classical pathway of complement, (2) targeting of microorganisms (opsonins) for phagocytosis by neutrophils and macrophages, and (3) targeting virally-infected cells for destruction by antibody-dependent cell-mediated immunity (ADCC). IgG antibodies are also critical to fetal immunity because they cross the placenta. IgE plays a role in parasite immunity and is also responsible for allergic reactions and anaphylactic shock. IgD is present on the membranes of B cells expressing monomeric IgM, although the role of IgD remains a mystery. IgM is the first antibody secreted in primary immune responses, and is involved in the activation of the classical component of complement. IgM antibodies are natural isohemagglutinins recognizing antigens of the ABO blood group present on erythrocytes. IgA is in mucosal secretions (e.g., tears, saliva, and colostrum of nursing mothers), and monomeric and dimeric IgA are secreted by plasma cells in mucosa-associated lymphoid tissue (MALT).

Antigen/antibody complexes precipitate out of solution after cross-linking of antibodies with multivalent antigens. When they are too big to remain soluble, the complexes undergo precipitation. Clumping or agglutination of immune complexes occurs when antibodies are cross-linked in certain proportions that favor that process, but neither cross-linking nor agglutination will happen if the antigen or antibody is present in excess. Also some particulate antigens have intrinsic negative charges, and when suspended in saline solution, an electrical potential called zeta potential is made that precludes articles from coming close together.

Antibodies secreted by plasma cells derived from a single B cell clone are called monoclonal, and they are produced in *biological factories* created by making hybridomas. These hybridomas are hybrid cells made from fusion of a normal spleen plasma cell and a malignant myeloma cell no longer secreting antibodies.

REVIEW OF KEY TERMS AND ABBREVIATIONS

Matching: Match the key term in the left column with the definition in the right column.

1. _____ specificity

2. _____ opsonization

3. _____ perforin

4. _____ secretory component

5. _____ zeta potential

6. _____ immunoglobulins

7. _____ differentiation

8. _____ electrophoresis

a) induce osmotic lysis of infected cell

b) relatively smaller protein chain with "V" & "J" segments

c) specialized or transformed (as B cells to plasma cells)

d) component of antibodies not changing

e) protein separation under influence of an electric field

f) prevents particles from coming close together

g) component of antibody providing its specificity

h) two antibody fragments that bind to antigen

9. _____ gamma globulins

i) refers to antibody recognizing a precise antigen segment

10. _____ light chains

j) proteins migrating closest to the anode

11. _____ variable region

k) antibodies; proteins with a major role in immunity

12. _____ constant region

l) antibody binding to a similar, not identical epitope

13. _____ bifunctional

m) phagocytosis following binding to an opsonin

14. _____ Fc fragment

n) does not bind antigen; readily crystallized

15. _____ Fab

o) epithelial receptor to which dimeric IgA antibody binds

16. _____ cross-reactivity

p) antibodies have two domains with separate functions

17. _____ avidity

q) association constant between antibody/univalent antigen

18. _____ affinity

r) minor differences in heavy chain constant region

19. _____ isotypes

s) measure of overall binding; antibody/epitope

20. _____ allotypes

t) mucosa-associated lymphoid tissues

21. _____ MALT

u) antibody classes; five heavy chain constant regions

Definitions: Write the definition of each of the following words or terms.

1. Bifunctional _____

   _____

2. Electrophoresis _____

   _____

3. Hybridoma _____

   _____

4. Isotypes _____

   _____

5. Monoclonal _____

_____

6. Variable Region _____

_____

7. Constant Region _____

_____

8. Affinity _____

_____

9. Avidity _____

_____

10. Antibody _____

_____

11. Cross-Reactivity _____

_____

12. Differentiation _____

_____

13. Major Basic Protein _____

_____

REVIEW EXERCISES

True or False: Read each statement and decide if it is TRUE or FALSE. Place T or F on the line before each statement.

1. _____ Proteins expressed on the surface of B cells are typically referred to as antibodies; and when they are secreted they are referred to as membrane immunoglobulin (mIg).

2. _____ Separation of proteins while under the influence of an electric field is called electrophoresis.

3. _____ The terms light chain and heavy chain refer to equal-sized proteins with constant and variable regions more or less identical.

4. _____ Each monomeric antibody has two identical antigen binding sites based on the combined variable regions of the light and heavy chains.

5. _____ The cross-reactivity property of antibodies has been exploited in the use of tetanus toxoid immunization to protect individuals ultimately from tetanus toxin.

Fill in the Blank: Complete the following sentences on the immune system by filling in the missing word or words.

1. Avidity is a measure of the overall binding between the antigen binding sites and multivalent _____ .

2. _____ is the association constant between antibody and a univalent antigen.

3. When some particulate antigens that have intrinsic negative charges are suspended in saline, an electric potential or _____ potential is generated, which precludes particles from getting close together.

4. _____ are antibody classes based on the five heavy chain constant regions.

5. Recognition sites for phagocytes are part of molecules deposited onto the antigen; the molecules are called _____ .

Multiple Choice: Choose the best answer.

1. Plasma cells secrete _____ rather than expressing them on the cell surface.

   a. isotypes
   b. secretory component
   c. serum
   d. allotypes
   e. immunoglobulins

2. Becoming specialized or transformed into plasma cells like B cells after activation by antigens is called

   a. cross-reactivity.
   b. differentiation.
   c. bifunctionality.
   d. susceptibility.
   e. avidity.

3. Secreted antibodies can be separated from other serum proteins by incorporating them within a supporting medium like polyacrylamide and exposing them to an electric field; this separation of proteins under the influence of an electric field is called

   a. differentiation.
   b. specificity.
   c. cross reactivity.
   d. avidity.
   e. electrophoresis.

4. Because antibodies have both an antigen-binding site and a separate domain determining other biological activities, they are said to be

   a. bifunctional.
   b. specific.
   c. cross reactive.
   d. soluble.
   e. precipitated.

5. In order to have antibodies specific for one epitope called _____ , it is necessary to immortalize normal spleen plasma cells into biological factories secreting antibodies of one specificity.

   a. monoclonal
   b. HAT
   c. PEG
   d. hybridoma
   e. perforin

CRITICAL THINKING EXERCISES

Critical Thinking 1: Read this scenario and then answer the questions that follow.

Some students are talking about lockjaw in the hall between classes, and they are confused about what it is since the lecture was given in microbiology, and how immunization works against it. Some of the comments made by the students are "I thought bacterial infection meant bacteria invaded and killed cells, so how can a 'toxoid' protect you from that?" and "Toxoids are poisons, aren't they? So, how can a poison help you fight off infection when you're already being poisoned?"

1. How would you explain to your confused friends what the specific problem with bacteria causing lockjaw is since you have taken immunology? Tell them how this particular bacterium works.

2. The confusion that the students have with the term "toxoid" and "toxin" seems to be a major source of their misunderstanding. How would you distinguish them?

3. Since you have taken immunology, take a moment to reflect on neutralization of antigens and explain to the students in the hall what cross-reactivity has to do with all this.

Critical Thinking 2: Read this scenario and then answer the questions that follow.

Tom is discussing antibodies with Sarah and Kim, and he mentions that they are made up of four polypeptide chains with constant and variable regions. Tom also says variable regions determine the specificity. Furthermore, Tom mentions B cells secreting antibodies in the first place; he says this is fundamentally all Sarah and Kim need to know for the up-coming quiz.

1. While Tom has not mentioned anything absolutely incorrect, he has left a whole lot of material out that was in the chapter. What would Sarah and Kim also need to know about those four polypeptide chains that Tom neglected to mention?

2. Tom mentions that B cells secrete antibodies, but has he forgotten to say "the rest of the story" about what happens to B cells in order to do that? What has Tom not told Kim and Sarah about this process?

3. What else has Tom not told Sarah and Kim about antibodies and their functions? He mentioned specificity, but what about something else antibodies do?

Critical Thinking 3: Read this scenario and then answer the questions that follow.

Sarah and Kim's classmates are studying just before a major test on antibodies, and the group is covering bifunctionality as a concept. Someone blurts out that antibody fragments were discovered by using a plant extract used in cooking sometimes to marinate meats and also by using a gastric enzyme. Another student says that a way to remember the fragments is to recall the name of a laundry detergent. Still a third student mentions that affinity and avidity are too similar to distinguish, so why bother.

1. What could Kim and Sarah say to clear up the affinity and avidity question, since they well know they are different concepts? Are there clear examples of the differences?

2. What gastric enzyme and plant extract are referred to by one of the students? What else do they need to look at about these fragments, and what is the significance?

3. What are the antibody fragments that the group is talking about, and what are their roles in antibody bifunctionality?

CASE STUDY

Kim's Aunt Margaret is Rh–, and Aunt Margaret is expecting her second child. Kim brings up the good news in the cafeteria at school one day soon after the immunology class has just finished the chapter on immunology.

1. Sarah wants to ask Kim a few questions, since she seems to remember some very important aspect about antibodies, Rh antigens, and pregnancy. What sorts of things might Sarah want to ask Kim concerning Aunt Margaret's pregnancy?

2. What are the beneficial aspects of antibodies and pregnancy that Kim may know and may have passed on as information to Aunt Margaret?

3. What is the possible outcome for Aunt Margaret's pregnancy, and what precautions might she have already taken on her physician's advice?

CHAPTER 4

CELLS AND TISSUES
OF INNATE IMMUNITY

OUTLINE

OBJECTIVES

Upon completion of this chapter, the reader should be able to:

1. Describe the role of primary and secondary lymphoid tissues in immunity.
2. Describe the role of phagocytes.
3. Describe how phagocytes interact with their antigenic targets.
4. Explain how pathogens are destroyed in the phagocytic vacuole.
5. Describe how phagocytes participate in immune complex clearance.
6. Explain the role of antigen presenting cells and why the dendritic cell is the "best."
7. Describe how natural killer cells recognize and destroy their targets.
8. Understand the role of eosinophils in helminth infection.
9. Understand the role of mast cells and basophils in inflammation.
10. Describe in general terms the approaches used to measure phagocyte and natural killer cell function.

SUMMARY OF KEY POINTS

Lymphocytes undergo maturation, differentiation, and proliferation in lymphoid organs like the bone marrow, thymus, spleen, MALT, and cutaneous immune system. B cells complete maturation in bone marrow, and T cells mature in the thymus after being derived from precursor cells in the bone marrow. The bone marrow and thymus both are referred to as primary lymphoid organs and the others are called secondary lymphoid tissues in which adaptive immune responses occur during first exposure to an antigen. After initial exposure and response, immune responses may occur at the site of infection.

Macrophages and neutrophils are phagocytic, interacting with, and ingesting microorganisms after recognition using primitive pattern recognition receptors (PPRR). These phagocytes interact with pathogens indirectly through opsonins. Opsonins interact with the phagocyte receptors and ingestion of the antigen proceeds into the phagosome. Lysosomal enzymes, reactive oxygen intermediates, and nitric oxide in the phagosomes are the *weapons* used to destroy the ingested microbes.

Natural killer cells play a role in host defense against viral infections, and these cells destroy cells infected with viruses. Some cancer cells have been shown to be eliminated by natural killer cells as well.

Parasitic infections, especially helminths, are destroyed by eosinophils. Eosinophils bind to the Fc region of IgE antibodies that are bound to helminths, and then release proteins (major basic protein and eosinophil cationic protein) toxic to helminths.

Two populations of inflammatory cells are mast cells and basophils with surface receptors for complement proteolytic fragments C3a, C4a, and C5a. When these receptors are engaged, the mast cells are said to degranulate; mast cells also degranulate in response to crosslinking between antigen and IgE which is bound to FceR present on both mast cells and basophils. Histamine, released during degranulation, increases vascular permeability, allowing circulating immune cells to enter infected tissue.

Defects in immune cells can be assessed by enumeration of the actual number of cells, and also by measuring immune cell function. Immune mechanisms in host defense can be understood by these tests.

REVIEW OF KEY TERMS AND ABBREVIATIONS

Matching: Match the key term in the left column with the definition in the right column.

1. _____ allergies

2. _____ anaphylatoxins

3. _____ anaphylaxis

4. _____ antigen presenting cells

5. _____ asthma

6. _____ autocrine

7. _____ basophils

8. _____ bursa equivalent

9. _____ chemotactic

10. _____ cytokines

11. _____ defensins

12. _____ dendritic cells

13. _____ eosinophil

14. _____ follicles

15. _____ germinal centers

16. _____ hematopoiesis

17. _____ histamine

18. _____ hydrogen peroxide

19. _____ hydroxyl radicals

20. _____ immune complexes

21. _____ interleukins

a) very exaggerated hypersensitivity reaction

b) makes small blood vessels leaky

c) cells like Langerhan's cells with long extensions

d) OH; cytotoxic for microorganisms

e) macrophage-derived cytokines

f) H_2O_2; cytotoxic for microorganisms

g) permeabilize some bacterial and fungal membranes

h) less exaggerated hypersensitivity responses

i) sites B cells undergo differentiation proliferation

j) bone marrow in humans; site of B cell maturation

k) activated macrophages secrete these

l) main defense in response to parasitic infections

m) innate immunity cells originate in this process

n) dendritic cells, macrophages, B cells

o) antigen-antibody together activate complement

p) said of molecules that attract cells

q) a type of hypersensitivity with bronchial constriction

r) within outer cortex; sites of B cells in lymph nodes

s) said of secretions affecting same cell as produced them

t) when activated they degranulate and release histamine

u) C3a, C4a, C5a bind mast cells, induce histamine release

Definitions: Write the definition of each of the following words or terms.

1. Bursa of Fabricius _____

_____

2. cutaneous immune system _____

_____

3. eosinophil cationic protein _____

_____

4. interferon gamma _____

_____

5. keratinocytes _____

_____

6. killer inhibitory receptor _____

_____

7. Langerhan's cells _____

_____

8. lymph nodes _____

_____

9. lymphoid _____

_____

10. myeloid _____

_____

11. mast cells _____

_____

12. Peyer's patches _____

_____

13. phagolysosome _____

_____

REVIEW EXERCISES

True or False: Read each statement and decide if it is TRUE or FALSE. Place T or F on the line before each statement.

1. _____ Macrophages can serve as antigen presenting cells, but neutrophils cannot.

2. _____ Myeloid precursor cells give rise to mature B cells and pre-T cells.

3. _____ The bone marrow and the thymus are referred to as primary lymphoid organs.

4. _____ Neutrophils are recruited to the site of infection under the influence of chemotactic molecules.

5. _____ Phagocytes have no way of directly interacting with microorganisms.

Fill in the Blank: Complete the following sentences on the immune system by filling in the missing word or words.

1. Fusion of cytosolic lysosomes with a phagosome forms a chimeric vacuole called a

   _____ .

2. _____ are receptors on phagocytes that can interact directly with a microorganism and that recognize a wide array of molecules that may be present on the surface of a microorganism.

3. _____ refers to the consumption of oxygen and formation of reactive oxygen intermediates from NADPH oxidase in the phagosome membrane.

4. Only beneficial T cells survive what is referred to as the _____ process in which thymocytes that are not potentially beneficial to the host die in the thymus.

5. Interaction of the natural killer cell with the antibody triggers the release of _____ , a molecule that inserts into the infected cell's membrane where it polymerizes to form a pore causing osmotic lysis of the infected cell.

Multiple Choice: Choose the best answer.

1. All of the following are from myeloid precursor cells except
   a. neutrophils.
   b. basophils.
   c. B cells.
   d. monocytes.
   e. eosinophils.

2. All of the following are secondary lymphoid tissue except
   a. spleen.
   b. bone marrow.
   c. lymph nodes.
   d. thymus.
   e. b and d

3. T cells that are in the thymus are called

   a. thymocytes.
   b. T cell receptors.
   c. monocytes.
   d. MALT.
   e. immunoglobulins.

4. The lymphoid follicles are aggregated in one region of the gut and are referred to as

   a. Langerhan's cells.
   b. keratinocytes.
   c. Peyer's patches.
   d. natural killer cells.
   e. mast cells.

5. When antigen is contained within a vacuole in the cytoplasm of the phagocyte, the vacuole is called the

   a. phagolysosome.
   b. phagosome.
   c. lysosome.
   d. primitive pattern recognition receptors (PPRP).
   e. lysozyme.

CRITICAL THINKING EXERCISES:

Critical Thinking 1: Read this scenario and then answer the questions that follow.

There is confusion over what antigen presenting cells are in the study group after immunology one day. Tom says they are called dendritic cells and that is that, although some of the group including Sarah do not understand what that means.

1. What does Tom mean by dendritic cells? Explaining what they are may help clear up some understanding about what antigen presenting cells are.

2. How do you make sure Sarah understands what antigen presenting cells are? What other cells may be involved and why?

3. What are the special antigen presenting cells in the epidermis called?

Critical Thinking 2: Read this scenario and then answer the questions that follow.

Kim points out to Sarah and Tom that phagocytes can interact with microorganisms directly, although Tom only remembers indirect interaction through opsonins and says so.

1. Who is correct in the discussion above, Tom or Kim? Why?

2. What is the nature of direct interaction in this case? What other method is usual with phagocytes?

3. What are the opsonins Tom refers to, and what molecules are opsonins?

Critical Thinking 3: Read this scenario and then answer the questions that follow.

The nursing and allied health students are discussing the formed elements in blood and happen to mention the eosinophils as the least prevalent of the formed elements. One of the nursing students asks you about what you are learning in immunology about eosinophils.

1. What do you know about the origin of eosinophils? Why are eosinophils mentioned in immunology?

2. What special function does the eosinophil play in innate immunity?

3. What part does binding play in this whole scenario?

CASE STUDY

While reviewing the journals and periodicals at the local hospital you come across an article on a case of chronic granulomatous disease (CGD). While you remember something about CGD in this chapter, you are anxious to learn more. It may make a good report for class, especially since you are taking a class in human genetics, too.

1. What is CGD and why would it be a topic of interest in a genetics class?

2. What clinical test that your chapter mentions would be of particular interest here? How does it work, and what does it check for and why?

3. You read that infections are very serious and become life threatening with CGD. Why is that so, and what hope exists for the future?

CHAPTER 5

B CELLS

OUTLINE

OBJECTIVES

Upon completion of this chapter, the reader should be able to:

1. Describe the structure of B cell antigen receptor complex and the role of the various components.
2. Explain the key steps in the development of B cells from progenitor cells to mature cells.
3. Describe the key elements of a primary immune response and the role of helper T cells.
4. Understand the differences between a primary and a secondary B cell immune response.
5. Describe how B cell activation is turned off (regulated).

SUMMARY OF KEY POINTS

B cells or B lymphocytes (cells of adaptive immunity), which arise from precursor cells in myeloid tissue in the bone marrow, recognize and interact with antigens to produce antibody-secreting plasma cells. This differentiation of B cells results in some memory cells whose role will be immunosurveillance, but most of the activated B cells will differentiate into plasma cells that live a few days and then die.

Naïve mature bone cells all express B cell receptors (membrane-bound antibody or membrane immunoglobulin) made up of constant and variable regions on their two light chains and two heavy chains. Variable regions are composed of V, (D), and J segments and give the immunoglobulin its specificity. V, (D), and J segments are linked at the DNA level when DNA is "cut and pasted" in somatic recombination. Specific DNA segments V, (D), and J are put together and the rest of the DNA segments are removed permanently. Uniqueness of the variable regions is due to addition or removal of nucleotides in which these segments are brought together. Some resulting B cell receptors will recognize self-proteins and thus be autoreactive, causing autoimmune reactions. To avoid this unpleasant eventuality these B cell receptors are eliminated via tolerance induction.

Alternative splicing is a phenomenon whereby naïve B cells express both IgM and IgD in their B cell receptor complexes, and only affects the constant region. Both IgM and IgD have the same specificity, therefore some naïve B cells after leaving the bone marrow will seed peripheral lymphoid tissues, and others will circulate in immunosurveillance.

Primary response follows activation of B cells to an initial antigen. With a T-dependent antigen the primary response includes the naïve B cell encountering the antigen, receiving appropriate T cell help, and then clonally expanding. Some clonal B cells will differentiate into IgM-secreting cells or plasma cells. Other clonal B cells will switch the isotype of the B cell receptor, and their antibodies will switch from mu and delta isotypes to express gamma, alpha, or epsilon heavy chain constant regions. This activation phenomenon is referred to as isotype switching.

Affinity maturation or somatic mutation is another phenomenon that occurs following isotype switching. Spontaneous mutations occur in the variable region of the membrane antibody, and those B cells whose antibody receptors have a higher affinity for the antigen are selected to live. After isotype switching and affinity maturation, some B cells will then differentiate into plasma cells secreting antibodies of the new isotype, and others will become memory cells.

B cell responses are primary (first exposure) in which there is a gradual increase in serum concentration of IgM reaching a peak seven to ten days after immunization, and secondary (subsequent exposure) in which the response is faster and of greater magnitude and which activates memory B cells to differentiate to plasma cells as well as a few naïve B cells.

Isotype switching or memory cell formation does not occur with B cell activation from T-independent antigens. Signals derived from T cells are necessary to trigger isotype switching and memory cell formation. Mitogens or polyclonal activators like lipopolysaccharide, Staphylococcus protein A, and pokeweed mitogen trigger proliferation of large numbers of B cells without regard to specificity of membrane-bound antigen. These mitogens can be enumerated by analysis of whole peripheral blood using flow cytometry, while B cell function can be determined by measuring total serum antibody or by the reverse hemolytic plaque assay.

REVIEW OF KEY TERMS AND ABBREVIATIONS

Matching: Match the key term in the left column with the definition in the right column.

1. _____ affinity maturation

2. _____ allelic exclusion

3. _____ alternative splicing

4. _____ anergic

5. _____ differentiation

6. _____ chimeric gene

7. _____ clonal expansion

8. _____ diversity

9. _____ DNA polymerase

10. _____ isotype switching

11. _____ memory cells

12. _____ monomeric IgM

13. _____ panmarker

14. _____ plasma cells

15. _____ somatic mutation

16. _____ specificity

a) chimeric gene disallows a chimeric gene on other allele

b) polysaccharides

c) when immature B cells express self-reactive IgM

d) initial encounter with antigen

e) expressed at all stages of B cell development

f) antibody _____ ; what constitutes the B cell repertoire

g) memory cells activated following encounter with antigen

h) CD 19 regulates B cell _____

i) immunosurveillance; higher avidity for antigen

j) unresponsive to further stimulation

k) each B cell within the clone has the same _____

l) protein antigens

m) refers to the spontaneous mutations in variable regions

n) change in constant region of an antibody molecule

o) is constructed by selection of one "V," one "D," one "J"

p) antibody secreting cells

17. _____ T-dependent antigen

    q) primary RNA spliced; mRNA encodes mu or delta

18. _____ T-independent antigen

    r) terminal deoxynucleotidyl transferase

19. _____ tolerance induction

    s) proliferation leads to an increase in B cell clone

20. _____ primary response

    t) unique B cell receptors are this; on B cell surface

21. _____ secondary response

    u) another term for affinity maturation

Definitions: Write the definition of each of the following words or terms.

1. B cell maturation _____

_____

2. B cell receptor _____

_____

3. B cell repertoire _____

_____

4. lipopolysaccharide _____

_____

5. membrane-bound antibody _____

_____

6. pneumococcal polysaccharide _____

_____

7. polysaccharides _____

_____

8. somatic recombination _____

_____

9. B cell receptor encoding _____

_____

10. CD 19 _____

_____

11. CD 20 _____

_____

12. recombinases _____

_____

13. CD40 and CD40L _____

_____

REVIEW EXERCISES

True or False: Read each statement and decide if it is TRUE or FALSE. Place T or F on the line before each statement.

1. _____ Causative agent of pneumonia is a T-independent antigen.

2. _____ Mitogens trigger the proliferation of large numbers of B cells.

3. _____ Secondary responses are not necessarily more rapid responses.

4. _____ B cells can be enumerated by analysis of whole blood using flow cytometry.

5. _____ B cell receptors are membrane-bound antibody.

Fill in the Blank: Complete the following sentences on the immune system by filling in the missing word or words.

1. Some of the activated B cells will become _____ whose role will be immunosurveillance.

2. The expression of unique B cell receptors is the result of _____ that is a process in which segments of DNA are rearranged .

3. Insertion or deletion of nucleotides is mediated by a template independent _____ .

4. _____ is on the cell surface of all B cells as they begin "life."

5. When immature B cells with self-reactive IgM (B cell receptor) bind self-antigens they become _____ , which means unresponsive to further stimulation.

Multiple Choice: Choose the best answer.

1. Chimeric gene ensures that a chimeric gene will not be constructed on the other allele.

    a. tolerance induction
    b. diversity
    c. allelic exclusion
    d. clonal expansion
    e. isotype switching

2. Spontaneous mutations occur in DNA of the heavy chain and light chain chimeric genes encoding the variable regions.

    a. affinity maturation
    b. isotype switching
    c. allelic exclusion
    d. clonal expansion
    e. tolerance induction

3. The _____ of B cell responses refers to the change in serum antibody concentration over time following exposure to the antigen (immunization).

    a. affinity maturation
    b. allelic exclusion
    c. tolerance induction
    d. diversity
    e. kinetics

4. _____ immune responses are those in which memory cells are activated following encounter with antigen.

    a. Primary
    b. Secondary
    c. Tertiary
    d. Diversity
    e. Inactivation
    f. Crosslinking

5. When somatic recombination is activated, a _____ is constructed by randomly selecting one "V" segment, one "D" segment, and one "J" segment.

    a. chimeric gene
    b. B cell receptor
    c. plasma cell
    d. panmarker
    e. DNA polymerase

CRITICAL THINKING EXERCISES

Critical Thinking 1: Read this scenario and then answer the questions that follow.

Sarah, Kim, and Tom are wondering about how messages are being molecularly received and forwarded to create clones of B cells with the same receptors to recognize the same antigen. Tom thinks specificity is a result of "what works" or "doesn't work" in terms of binding antigen; while Sarah thinks that Tom's short summation explains some of it, she knows there is more. Kim is studying chemistry and genetics, and she has some answers for both Tom and Sarah.

1. What part of explaining specificity does Tom's comment make? Why is it too simple to explain what actually occurs?

2. What chemistry and genetics, supplied hopefully by Kim, are necessary to make the entire story clear for Sarah and Tom?

3. How many B cell receptors (antibodies) may be expressed on a B cell surface? When does the B cell acquire its receptor?

Critical Thinking 2: Read this scenario and then answer the questions that follow.

In autoimmune diseases like rheumatoid arthritis or lupus erythematosus, there are antibodies, which are self-reactive; that is, these antibodies recognize self. In this chapter students learn how these self-reactive IgM receptors are produced in the first place under normal conditions without any other genetic problem.

1. How are these self-reactive B cell receptors produced even under normal situations?

2. What processes are in place normally to deal with this eventuality of creating the V, (D), and J segments in construction of variable regions of light and heavy chains such that the variable regions recognize self?

3. When the autoimmune disease strikes, what do you think has to happen for its self-reactive antibodies to wreak continual havoc? (In other words, what goes wrong other than the obvious genetics problem?) What might be a solution?

CASE STUDY

An acquaintance of yours is mentioning that she has had the same illness twice within a year, but that the second time around was a lot less severe in signs and symptoms than the first time encountering the "bug." Since the acquaintance knows you are studying immunology, and she also wants to understand what has happened to lessen her symptoms. She's hoping you can tell her what has happened.

1. What background would you give your acquaintance to help her understand what happens in her body when it encounters a "bug" and why?

2. Compare primary and secondary antibody responses so your acquaintance might see what has happened to lessen the symptoms and signs the second time around. (Lag time, IgM and IgG serum titer changes, and magnitude of response are all-important parts of this puzzle.)

3. What cells are critical to figuring this scenario out? Why?

CHAPTER 6

THE MAJOR HISTOCOMPATIBILITY COMPLEX, ANTIGEN PROCESSING, AND ANTIGEN PRESENTATION

OUTLINE

- Recognition of Non-Self
- Major Histocompatibility Complex
  - Class I MHC in Humans
  - Class II MHC in Humans
  - Role of MHC in Immune Responses
- MHC Genes and Disease
  - Relative Risk and Hypotheses
- Transplantation
  - Graft Rejection
  - Immunosuppressive Therapies
  - Screening to Ensure Compatibility
- Antigen Processing and Antigen Presentation
  - Antigen Processing and Presentation with Class I MHC
  - Antigen Processing and Presentation with Class II MHC

OBJECTIVES

Upon completion of this chapter, the reader should be able to:

1. Explain how T cells and B cells recognize antigens.
2. Discuss the major histocompatibility complex (MHC) from a historical perspective.
3. List the three forms of class I MHC and three forms of class II MHC molecules.
4. Understand the concept of polymorphism and why it is advantageous to a population.
5. Explain the nomenclature used to refer to the numerous allelic variants of each MHC form.
6. List the various allelic forms of MHC and the disease susceptibility that these confer.
7. Discuss the various hypotheses put forth to explain the correlation between disease susceptibility and distinct MHC alleles.
8. Explain the differences between tissue matching and tissue typing.
9. Describe how exogenous antigens are processed and then displayed on the cell surface in association with class II MHC.
10. Describe how endogenous antigens are processed and then displayed on the cell surface in association with class I MHC.

SUMMARY OF KEY POINTS

T cells recognize antigen fragments (peptides) bound to antigen-presenting molecules and then displayed on the cell surface. Antigen-presenting molecules are encoded by various genes called the major histocompatibility complex. Two classes of antigen-presenting molecules, class I MHC and class II MHC, have several distinct allelic forms.

Using genetic techniques to study tissue rejection, the MHC region was first discovered by scientists in mice. The sera from individuals who received blood transfusions (foreign graft) and mothers having more than one pregnancy (multiparous) who received fetal cells during delivery (foreign graft) allowed identification of the MHC in humans. The sera from these individuals were used to assess ability of antibodies to lyse cells from other individuals.

Because MHC molecules were antigens present already on human leukocytes, these proteins were also referred to as human leukocyte antigens (HLAs), and the gene locus that encoded them was referred to as the HLA locus. The HLA locus is therefore called the MHC locus, the generic term used for this locus in all species, and the terms HLA and MHC are used interchangeably.

Serological studies revealed three genes, HLA-A, HLA-B, and HLA-C, and HLA-D from the human class II MHC region that were identified because lymphocytes from genetically disparate individuals proliferate when cultured together. This reaction is called a mixed lymphocyte reaction (MLR). B cell and monocyte research also revealed that the HLA-D region had three gene loci (P, Q, and R). All the HLA genes (A, B, C, DP, DQ, and DR) have many variant (allelic) forms in the population, so the HLA genes are said to be polymorphic and each allele is given a number. Epidemiological studies have shown that the HLA allele an individual inherits predisposes that individual to certain diseases.

Histocompatibility testing is performed via tissue matching (in which the goal is determining whether the tissue from one individual will be rejected when transplanted into another individual) and tissue typing (in which the individual's genotype is determined).

T cell activation is based on recognition of antigen peptides on the cell surface in association with MHC. CD4+ T cells recognize antigen presented with class II MHC, while CD8+ T cells recognize antigen presented with class I MHC. Class II MHC expression is limited to antigen-presenting cells and only these cells display antigen peptides to CD4+ T cells, while all nucleated cells express class I MHC and any one of these cells has the potential to display antigen peptides to CD8+ cells.

REVIEW OF KEY TERMS AND ABBREVIATIONS

Matching: Match the key term in the left column with the definition in the right column.

1. _____ allelic

a) cytosolic vesicle

2. _____ allografts

b) grafts across species

3. _____ chronic rejection

c) each person has unique pattern of fragmentation

4. _____ class I MHC

d) goal is to match donor and recipient as to MHC compatibility

5. _____ class II MHC

e) classified as hyperacute, acute, or chronic

6. _____ codominant

f) gene region on chromosome 6; encodes AP molecules

7. _____ cross-reactive

g) said of a gene with many variant forms in population

8. _____ endosome

h) forms are HLA-A, HLA-B, and HLA-C

9. _____ genotype

i) allows direct amplification of DNA sequence

10. _____ graft rejection

j) one hypothesis for autoimmune reactivity

11. _____ haplotype

k) sum of the haplotypes

12. _____ isograft

l) determine the HLA alleles on individual's leukocytes

13. _____ MHC

m) the variant forms for a gene in the population

14. _____ molecular mimicry

n) multi-enzyme complex degrades proteins with ubiquitin

15. _____ PCR

o) no genetic difference between donor and recipient

16. _____ polymorphic

p) grafts between members of the same species

17. _____ proteasome

q) epitopes stimulus for immune responses and disease

18. _____   RFLP

19. _____   tissue matching

20. _____   tissue typing

21. _____   xenograft

r) alleles of each parent are expressed on each cell

s) set of MHC alleles from one parent

t) occurs weeks, months, or years post transplant

u) helper T cells cannot be activated in their absence

Definitions: Write the definition of each of the following words or terms.

1. MHC _____

_____

2. class I MHC _____

_____

3. MLR _____

_____

4. linkage disequilibrium _____

_____

5. GvHD _____

_____

6. RFLPs _____

_____

7. PCR _____

_____

8. TAP proteins _____

_____

9. endosomes _____

_____

10. class II MHC _____

_____

11. genotype _____

_____

12. polymorphic _____

_____

13. allelic _____

_____

REVIEW EXERCISES

True or False: Read each statement and decide if it is TRUE or FALSE. Place T or F on the line before each statement.

1. _____   Class I MHC molecules are made up of two polypeptides; a polymorphic heavy chain and a non-polymorphic light chain.

2. _____   The MHC gene region is located on chromosome 15 in humans.

3. _____   For class II MHC each HLA (A, B, C) gene has many variant forms in the population.

4. _____   The human class II MHC region was identified using the mixed lymphocyte reaction (MLR).

5. _____   Each of the three forms of class I MHC molecules are codominantly expressed.

Fill in the Blank: Complete the following sentences on the immune system by filling in the missing word or words.

1. The association with HLA and disease may not be limited to predisposition to disease, but also influence disease _____ .

2. A variation of the molecular mimicry theme suggests that _____ epitopes, and not identical epitopes, serve as the stimulus for immunological responses and disease.

3. Genes are said to be in _____ when two genes are inherited together in higher frequency than would be predicted from chance.

4. _____ are grafts in which there is no genetic difference between the donor and recipient.

5. In _____ the main rejection is that of the graft rejecting all the recipient tissues.

Multiple Choice: Choose the best answer.

1. The MHC is a gene region located on chromosome

   a. 15.
   b. 6.
   c. H-2.
   d. HLA-A.
   e. histocompatibility antigens.

2. The "culprits" in graft versus host disease are

   a. recipient tissues.
   b. activated B cells.
   c. T cells.
   d. macrophages.
   e. cyclosporin A.

3. All the following are immunosuppressive therapies except

   a. cyclosporin A.
   b. FK 506.
   c. prednisone.
   d. cell-derived cytokines.
   e. antibodies targeting specific cell surface molecules on T cells.

4. The _____ is a simple, automated, rapid in vitro technique allowing direct amplification of a particular DNA sequence in the presence of primers bordering the gene of interest.

   a. RFLP
   b. MLR
   c. PCR
   d. MHC
   e. TAP

CRITICAL THINKING EXERCISES

Critical Thinking 1: Read this scenario and then answer the questions that follow.

Sarah and Kim are talking about MHC genes and disease in preparation for an informal seminar they're giving next week for the nursing class. Sarah is of the opinion that the genetic predisposition explains it all and she is preparing a chart to demonstrate that point, while Kim wants a balanced view of all research so far and wants to discuss viable hypotheses.

1. What sorts of things will appear on Sarah's chart? What relative risks will appear? What could account for all the "rest of the story"?

2. What kinds of things will Kim want to bring up to explain associations of particular diseases with a given allele?

3. How useful is this debate on association with disease and alleles? Why or why not is the debate useful?

Critical Thinking 2: Read this scenario and then answer the questions that follow.

At a health fair at your school the allied health department is discussing burns, and how grafts are used to conserve body fluids and prevent infection. A few nursing students want the frame of reference that you gained from immunology. While you mention genetic disparity, they are talking more about burn severity and "fixes."

1. What is the difference between the views that the nurses may have from their perspective and your outlook from immunology?

2. What eventually negates the differences between you and the nursing students about grafts? Why?

3. What determines the most vigorous rejection episodes? What might be done to promote graft success initially and after the graft?

CASE STUDY

An infamous paternity suit is all the rage in the local newspapers. Some of the histocompatibility tests you have heard about in immunology class have been referred to in the news. Since almost every test has been rejected on some legal grounds or other, you are very interested in reviewing the science. Also, a relative of yours asks you about the news and what is accurate and what is not.

1. What sorts of tests would be included in this case?

2. What would these histocompatibility tests determine or not? Why or why not?

3. What is the primary science involved here, regardless of the "legal grounds?"

CHAPTER 7

T CELLS

OUTLINE

- T cells
- General Features of T cell Receptors
  - T cell Repertoire
- T cell Maturation
  - Somatic Recombination and Construction of T cell receptors
  - Allelic Exclusion
  - Tolerance Induction
- CD4+ T cells Encounter Antigen
  - Antigen Presentation to CD4+ T cells
  - Signals Required for Activation of CD4+ T cells
  - T cell Growth Factor
  - Fate of Activated CD4+ Naïve T cells
  - T cell Cytokines in Host Defense
  - Fate of Activated CD4+ T cells
- CD8+ T cells
  - Activation and Differentiation of pCTL to CTL
  - Destruction of Infected Cells
  - Fate of CD8+ T cells
- Memory T cells
- Enumeration of T cells
- Approaches for the Isolation of T cells
  - Magnetic Beads for Separation of Cells
  - Cell Sorting for Separation of Cells

- ■ Complement Fixation for Removal of Cells
- ■ Miscellaneous Approaches
- ■ Assessing T cell Function
  - ■ Cell Proliferation

OBJECTIVES

Upon completion of this chapter, the reader should be able to:

1. Describe the structure of T cell antigen receptor complex and the role of the various components.
2. Explain the role of somatic recombination during T cell maturation in the thymus.
3. Explain the selection process by which T cells are eliminated if they are of no value to the host, or if they are potentially autoreactive.
4. Explain what is meant by lineage commitment.
5. Explain the role of antigen-presenting cells in T cell activation.
6. Name the cytokines whose presence determines whether Th1 or Th2 cells will develop from activated Thp cells.
7. Understand why the secretion of Type 1 versus Type 2 cytokines secretion affects immunity.
8. Explain why pCTL cannot deliver a lethal hit and the requirements for their development to mature CTL capable of killing their target cell.
9. Describe how a CTL kills virally-infected cells.
10. Describe how T cells are enumerated, isolated, and how function is assessed.

SUMMARY OF KEY POINTS

While playing a central role in immune responses, T cells and their immune responses depend on the subclass to which they belong. T helper cells (Th) secrete cytokines necessary to other cells to carry out their function in immune responses. Killer or cytotoxic T cells destroy infected cells displaying an antigen fragment complexed with class I MHC on the cell surface. Each T cell clone has a unique receptor on its surface capable of recognizing an antigen/MHC complex.

Two transmembrane polypeptide chains called alpha and beta make up the T cell receptors, with each chain consisting of a variable and a constant region. The variable region, composed of segments, is what makes the receptor so unique. Addition or deletion of nucleotides at the segment junction and the combination of alpha and beta chains generate T cell receptors recognizing a wide array of antigen/MHC complexes.

T cell receptors also are expressed that may be of no value, or worse, autoreactive. Cells expressing these receptors are eliminated during maturation in the thymus by processes called death by neglect and negative selection. Those T cells with potentially beneficial receptors are positively selected. After selection these T cells undergo a developmental stage in which they will express either CD4 or CD8, and correlates with the immunological function of the T cell. The role of CD4+ T cells is cytokine secretion, while the role of CD8+ T cells is destruction of infected cells. The class of cytokines will also determine the course of an infectious disease because Type 1 cytokines support cell-mediated immunity while Type 2 cytokines support humoral immune responses. After infection, some T cells will become memory T cells and function in immunosurveillance, but most of the activated T cells die.

Immunodeficiency disorders can be diagnosed with enumeration of T cells in peripheral blood. Many assays require isolation of mononuclear cells from blood components, followed by removal of non-T cells or by further isolation of T cells. To target T cells, antibodies specific for a protein (marker) on T cells bind to T cells and serve as the marker for identifying the T cells. CD2 and CD3 are pan-markers for T cells, while CD4 and CD8 serve as markers for subpopulations of T cells. Rosetting techniques can also be used to separate T cells from other mononuclear cells. T cells bind to sheep red blood cells (SRBC), where the SRBC form a rosette around the T cell.

CD8+ T cell function can be assessed based on the ability of activated T cells to bind to a target cell, and secrete molecules that induce osmotic lysis of that target cell. These target cells are incubated with radioactive chromium, and then lysed by toxic molecules secreted by the activated T cells, releasing radiolabeled chromium, which can be measured to assess CD8+ T cell cytolytic function.

CD4+ T cell function can be assessed by cytokine secretion. One of the cytokines, IL-2, is a growth factor for T cells, so an assessment of CD4+ T cell function can be made in vitro by measuring clonal expansion (proliferation) of IL-2 dependent cells in response to incubation with culture medium from polyclonally activated CD4+ T cells.

REVIEW OF KEY TERMS AND ABBREVIATIONS

Matching: Match the key term in the left column with the definition in the right column.

1. _____ AIDS

a) T cell receptor

2. _____ helper T cells

b) growth factor, as autocrine and paracrine

3. _____ cytotoxic T cells

c) processes of the T cell arriving to the thymus

4. _____ TCR

d) most recent techniques for T cell isolation

5. _____ T cell repertoire

e) perform "cutting and pasting" of the DNA

6. _____ T cell maturation

f) T cells and CD2 form these with RBCs, LFA-3

7. _____ adhesion molecule

g) initial screening of thymocyte interaction with this

8. _____ recombinases

h) acquired immunodeficiency disorder syndrome

9. _____ death by neglect

i) after antigen is gone, most T cells die this way

10. _____ negative selection

j) CD2 required for stable cell/cell conjugation

11. _____ positive selection

k) insertion or deletion of nucleotides where V, D, J are

12. _____ Interleukin-2 (IL-2)

l) CD8+ T cells (destruction of infected host cells)

13. _____ interferon gamma

m) after second selection T cells circulate in this role

14. _____ programmed cell death

n) thymocytes recognizing self MHC too well

15. _____ memory cells

o) total number of T cell clones defines this

16. _____ rosettes

p) function of the flow cytometry to select

17. _____ magnetic beads

q) some Th1 and Th2 clones become dormant

18. _____ cell sorting

r) thymocytes not recognizing self MHC

19. _____ junctional diversity

s) cytokine secreted by activated natural killer cells and Th1

20. _____ thymic epithelium

t) CD4+ T cells (cytokine secretion)

21. _____ immunosurveillance

u) thymocytes with just the right avidity for self-MHC

Definitions: Write the definition of each of the following words or terms.

1. AIDS _____

_____

2. T cells _____

_____

3. TCR _____

_____

4. T cell maturation _____

_____

5. thymocyte _____

_____

6. somatic recombination _____

_____

7. recombinases _____

_____

8. chimeric gene _____

_____

9. T cell activation _____

_____

10. interferon gamma _____

_____

11. memory cells _____

_____

12. perforin _____

_____

13. isolation of T cells _____

_____

REVIEW EXERCISES

True or False: Read each statement and decide if it is TRUE or FALSE. Place T or F on the line before each statement.

1. _____   T cells contribute to humoral immunity.

2. _____   The primary role of CD8+ T cells is cytokine secretion.

3. _____   The T cell receptor is a heterodimer made up of three transmembrane polypeptide chains called alpha, beta, and delta.

4. _____   Each T cell within a clone does not necessarily have the same specificity.

5. _____   T cells recognize fragments of antigen complexed with a major histocompatibility complex protein displayed on the surface of cells.

Fill in the Blank: Complete the following sentences on the immune system by filling in the missing word or words.

1. It is the _____ (which along with the heterodimer makes up the T cell receptor) that interacts with the biochemical signaling pathways.

2. Numerous cell divisions are required to form a _____ of sufficient numbers of T cells.

3. The total number of T cell clones defines the T cell _____ .

4. T cell _____ refers to the processes that the progenitor T cell arriving to the thymus undergoes to become a mature T cell.

5. While in the thymus the developing T cell is often referred to as a _____ .

Multiple Choice: Choose the best answer.

1. The process whereby mature T cells are separated into functional subsets, the CD4+ helper T cells and the CD8+ cytotoxic T cells, is referred to as

   a. maturation.
   b. lineage determination.
   c. T cell repertoire.
   d. specificity.
   e. somatic recombination.

2. Special enzymes, termed _____ , perform the task of cutting and pasting the DNA when it is rearranged in the variable region of the T cell receptor.

   a. proteases
   b. IL-2
   c. interferon gamma
   d. deoxynucleotidyl transferase
   e. recombinases

3. Ensuring that a chimeric gene will not be constructed on the other allele is

   a. allelic exclusion.
   b. negative selection.
   c. death by neglect.
   d. positive selection.
   e. immunosurveillance.

4. The sentinel role of cells in host defense against microbial invasion is

   a. death by neglect.
   b. positive selection.
   c. avidity.
   d. affinity.
   e. immunosurveillance.

CRITICAL THINKING EXERCISES

Critical Thinking 1: Read this scenario and then answer the questions that follow.

Some members of the class are considering the maturation of T cells, the ensuing naïve T cells committed as they are to being either CD4+ or CD8+, and their subsequent activation. As confusing as the selection process seems in the thymus, the change from naïve to activated status is what is confusing most students, especially concerning CD4+ T cells and the two sorts of cytokines they will produce as Th1 cells and Th2 cells.

1. What general things could you say about naïve CD4+ T cell activation? And, what does naïve mean in this context exactly? (That may be another stumbling block.)

2. What do the two sorts of cytokines mediate in the immune process?

3. How would you explain a naïve CD4+ T cell becoming either a Th1 or Th2 but not both? (*Hint*: Think about the microenvironment. Why there are such differences in the way normal healthy individuals respond to the same infection could be partially answered by this.)

Critical Thinking 2: Read this scenario and then answer the questions that follow.

In discussing immune responses to infectious agents, a nursing student refers to the difference between responses to an initial encounter with an antigen and subsequent encounters. The nursing student simply says that the body "learns how to fight off the infectious agent more effectively." Tom and Sarah, hearing this comment, have to join into the conversation.

1. What do you think Tom and Sarah have to say to the remark made by the nursing student? Why do you think they must respond to it?

2. What differences can be cited between CD4+ T cells and CD8+ T cells in this scenario? What are the similarities?

3. Cite the time differences in initial and subsequent encounters with the infectious agent. What accounts for the initial time period?

CHAPTER 8

COMPLEMENT

OUTLINE

- Complement
- Classical Pathway of Complement
    - Components
    - Activation
- Alternative Pathway of Complement
    - Components
    - Activation
- Regulation of Complement
    - Regulation of Classical Pathway
    - Regulation of C3 Convertases
    - Regulation of Membrane Attack Complex
- Complement Receptors
- Biological Activities of Complement
    - Role of Complement in the Inflammatory Response
    - Role of Complement in Phagocytosis
    - Role of Complement in the Elimination of Immune Complexes
    - Role of Complement in Osmotic Lysis of Bacteria
    - Evading the Biological Activities of Complement
- Complement Deficiencies and Disease
    - C1 Inhibitor Protein Deficiency
    - Deficiencies in C2 and C4
    - Deficiencies in Membrane Linkage for Regulatory Proteins
    - Deficiencies in MAC Proteins
    - Deficiencies in C3

- ■ Evaluating Complement Pathways
  - ■ Measurement of Overall Complement Activity
  - ■ Measurement of Complement Components

OBJECTIVES

Upon completion of this chapter, the reader should be able to:

1. Describe the components of the classical pathway of complement and the role of the various components.
2. Describe the components of the alternative pathway of complement and the role of the various components.
3. Understand how the activation of the classical pathway of complement differs from that of the alternative pathway.
4. Explain how complement regulatory proteins protect the host cells from the damaging effects of complement.
5. Describe the various biological activities of complement in host defense.
6. Explain the consequences of deficiencies in various components of the complement cascade or regulatory proteins.
7. Describe the basic principles of tests that are used to evaluate the overall activity of the classical and alternative pathways.
8. Explain the difference in tests that measure overall complement activity with those tests that measure the activity of individual complement components

SUMMARY OF KEY POINTS

Complement is a system of proteins playing a major role in host defense. Some proteins are in the circulation, and other proteins of the complement system are membrane bound. Two pathways may activate complement; one that is referred to as the classical pathway requires antibody, while the other is referred to as the alternative pathway and has no requirement for antibody. Activation of complement is called a cascade because many of the proteins are sequentially activated one after the other. Enzymatic complexes are assembled from some of the activated proteins such as C3 convertase and C5 convertase, which cleave C3 and C5 respectively. Fragments derived from this cleaving are important in host defense, as for example one of the fragments of C5 cleavage (C5b) combines with other proteins to form a complex, which makes a pore in cell (bacterial) membranes, destroying the integrity of the membrane so that the bacteria are destroyed by osmotic lysis. Some other complement proteins, outside of the cascade, serve to regulate the action of the activated proteins to protect autologous cells from damage.

Regulatory proteins for complement are in circulation and membrane bound, and protect host cells from possible damage from activation of complement in host defense. Complement is regulated via classical pathway activation, C3 convertases of both alternative and classical pathway, anaphylatoxins, and regulation of the membrane attack complex (MAC).

Deficiencies of complement components and regulatory proteins are seen, although these deficiencies are rare and usually inherited. Patients present with an increased tendency to infection, especially bacterial, as well as with an excessive immune complex deposition in tissues. Genetic and acquired angioedema is correlated with a deficiency in C1 inhibitor protein (C1 INH), and patients present with recurrent bouts of limited swelling of the face, extremities, and the gastrointestinal tract. Individuals with systemic lupus erythematosus (SLE) have deficiencies in C2 or C4 (early classical complement pathway proteins), and individuals presenting recurrent infections especially of *Neisseria sp.* may have deficiencies of complement proteins of the membrane attack complex (MAC) or Factor H, Factor I, and properdin (alternative pathway control proteins).

Most cells make two types of the regulatory protein DAF and CD59, some of which are attached to the cell surface via GPI linkages or some with transmembrane domains. Normal red blood cells express only DAF and CD59 with GPI linkage, so individuals unable to make the GPI linkage do not express the complement regulatory proteins on the red blood cell surface leading to lysis by complement and subsequent anemia referred to as paroxysmal nocturnal hemoglobinuria. Complement testing may be used to assess complement deficiencies or complement activation in immune complex associated diseases such as glomerulonephritis, rheumatoid arthritis, or systemic lupus erythematosus. Total classical complement pathway testing and MAC function may be assessed via the CH_{50} assay in an efficient and cost-effective way. Radioimmundiffusion based on immune complex precipitation in agar gels and rate nephelometry utilizing the light scattering property of light when it contacts a non-soluble particle are tests for specific complement components.

REVIEW OF KEY TERMS AND ABBREVIATIONS

Matching: Match the key term in the left column with the definition in the right column.

1. _____ classical pathway

2. _____ alternative pathway

3. _____ complement fixation

4. _____ anaphylatoxin

5. _____ C3 convertases

6. _____ MAC

7. _____ common pathway

8. _____ PNH

9. _____ CR1

10. _____ CR2

11. _____ CR3

12. _____ chemokines

13. _____ bradykinin

a) binds to receptors present on mast cells/basophils

b) radial immunodiffusion tests

c) chemokines attract cells to certain sites

d) receptor for complement fragment C3b

e) systemic lupus erythematosus

f) present on phagocytes and natural killer cells

g) C1 binds to IgM (or IgG) bound to bacterial cell

h) present on B cells; target for Epstein Barr Virus

i) molecules that cause the process of chemotaxis

j) both terminate with formation of MAC

k) induces vascular permeability

l) paroxysmal nocturnal hemoglobinuria

m) regulatory protein in alternative pathway

14. _____   SLE   n) pathway that requires antibody

15. _____ CH_{50} and AH_{50} o) membrane attack complex

16. _____   RID   p) regulatory protein of classical pathway

17. _____   nephelometry   q) measure overall complement activity

18. _____   properdin   r) utilizes light scattering property

19. _____   C1 inhibitor   s) enzymes which cleave C3

20. _____   chemotaxis   t) pathway independent of antibody

Definitions: Write the definition of each of the following words or terms.

1. complement _____

_____

2. classical pathway _____

_____

3. alternative pathway _____

_____

4. cascade _____

_____

5. complement fixation _____

_____

6. anaphylatoxin _____

_____

7. MAC _____

_____

8. properdin _____

_____

9. common pathway _____

_____

10. complement receptors _____

_____

11. degranulation _____

_____

12. chemokines _____

_____

13. bradykinin _____

_____

REVIEW EXERCISES

True or False: Read each statement and decide if it is TRUE or FALSE. Place T or F on the line before each statement.

1. _____ SLE is a systemic autoimmune disorder.

2. _____ Nephelometry is a technique that utilizes precipitation of immune complexes.

3. _____ Angioedema is associated with a deficiency in C1 INH.

4. _____ The causative agent of mononucleosis is the Epstein Barr virus.

Fill in the Blank: Complete the following sentences on the immune system by filling in the missing word or words.

1. _____ is a system of numerous proteins playing an important role in host defense.

2. The pathway requiring antibody is called the _____ pathway of complement.

3. The pathway independent of antibody is referred to as the _____ pathway of complement.

4. Some proteins functioning as regulatory proteins in the classical pathway of complement are _____ .

5. _____ stabilizes the alternative pathway C3 convertase.

Multiple Choice: Choose the best answer.

1. Inhibits MAC formation.

   a. C4 binding protein
   b. complement receptor type 1
   c. properdin
   d. factor I
   e. vitronectin

2. Prevents initiation of complement activation.

   a. C4 binding protein
   b. C1 inhibitor
   c. delay accelerating factor
   d. anaphylatoxin
   e. vitronectin

3. Cleaves and inactivates C3b and C4b.

   a. C4 binding protein
   b. C1 inhibitor
   c. properdin
   d. factor I
   e. anaphylatoxin

4. C1 binds to IgM or IgG that is bound to a bacterial cell surface.

   a. C1 inhibition
   b. C4 binding
   c. C5 convertase alternative pathway
   d. complement fixation
   e. terminal pathway

CRITICAL THINKING EXERCISES

Critical Thinking 1: Read this scenario and then answer the questions that follow.

An open debate has ensued in immunology class over all the regulatory proteins. Principally, the fundamental issue to the students is the fine line they perceive between activation and regulation. The two pathways are creating an issue for the students also, because of what seems so complex. One student says: "Regulatory proteins protect autologous cells, don't they?"

1. What are the regulatory proteins for complement? What are they essentially for? How do they affect complement? What are autologous cells?

2. What are the two complement pathways, and what is common and different about them? Why do you think the students in immunology class are confused about them?

3. How is complement regulated exactly? Does this shed light on the apparent complexity? Why or why not?

Critical Thinking 2: Read this scenario and then answer the questions that follow.

In human anatomy and physiology class you have heard how certain white blood cells leave the vascular compartment (the blood) in order to go into infected tissues. And then in immunology class you are exposed to the idea of complement and chemical processes that the complement system induces. You want to put these ideas together, since you know they must be connected.

1. What are some examples of certain white blood cells that exit the blood vessels to enter infected areas of the body? How do they do that?

2. What chemicals that you learned about in this chapter allow the white blood cells to leave the vascular compartment and be attracted to inflammatory sites?

3. What happens in the spleen and liver to red blood cells (with CR1 receptors on them such as neutrophils)?

CASE STUDY

A friend of yours is working at the hospital during the clinical aspect of a particular class for the nursing program at your school. You hear them talk about recurrent gonorrhea and meningitis, angioedema, and paroxysmal nocturnal hemoglobinuria. You are surprised to realize that although you are in another program of study altogether you understand what they are referring to in conversation because you are taking immunology.

1. What are recurrent gonorrhea and meningitis, angioedema, and PNH from your point of view?

2. How do you explain these disorders to your nursing friend?

3. What sorts of tests or assays may be used to screen for them?

CHAPTER 9

ORCHESTRATION OF HOST DEFENSES IN RESPONSE TO INFECTION

OUTLINE

- Orchestration of Host Defenses in Response to Infection
  - Challenge of Immunology
  - Challenge of Infectious Agents
- Infectious Agents Outside of Cells: Extracellular Microbes
  - Orchestration of Localized Host Defense Mechanisms in Primary Infections
  - Destination: Lymph Node
  - Memory Immune Responses
- Microbes That Thrive in Phagosomes
  - Orchestration of Host Defense Mechanisms in Primary Infections
- Microbes Present in the Cell Cytosol
  - Orchestration of Host Defenses in Primary Infections

OBJECTIVES

Upon completion of this chapter, the reader should be able to:

1. Discuss the role of the (i) alternative pathway of complement, (ii) mast cells and vascular endothelial cells, (iii) phagocytes, and (iv) antigen-presenting cells in host defense to infectious agents that are outside the cell.

2. Explain how the effector molecules generated via various host defense mechanisms integrate and enhance the efficacy of the other branch of the immune system during various types of infections.

3. Discuss the role of macrophages, CD4+ T cells, and Type 1 cytokines in host defense to infectious agents that thrive inside the phagosome.

4. Discuss the role of CD4+ T cells, Type 1 cytokines, pCTL, and CTL in host defense to infectious agents that thrive inside cytosol but are not contained within a vacuole.

5. Discuss the role of natural killer cells in viral immunity.

SUMMARY OF KEY POINTS

Like an orchestra with many instruments contributing to a music production, so the immune system with various cell types are recruited to produce an immune response. Infectious agents are in five major groups: extracellular bacteria, intracellular bacteria, viruses, parasites, and fungi. From the perspective of the location of the infectious agent, the complexity of host defense mechanisms can be simplified into three locations: outside the cell, inside a phagosome, or inside the cytoplasm.

Microbes in tissues but still outside the cell can be targeted by the following host defenses: alternative pathway of complement, mast cells and vascular endothelial cells, phagocytes, and antigen-presenting cells. Inflammation is the manifestation of these host defense mechanisms.

Microbes thriving in phagosomes are intracellular organisms, and several host defense mechanisms may resolve this type of infection but not in the absence of Type 1 cytokines. Type 1 cytokine interferon gamma (IFNγ, which enhances NADPH oxidase and induces nitric oxide synthase) is made by Th1 cells, and tumor necrosis factor (TNF) is made by both activated macrophages and Th1 cells. NADPH leads to more production of reactive oxygen intermediates and nitric oxide synthase catalyzes the reaction to make nitric oxide (NO). The specific role of TNF is not known, but NO formed in the cytosol of phagocytes may cross the membrane into the phagosome.

For the most part infectious agents in the cytosol but not contained within a phagosome are viruses, which are inaccessible to the many immune mechanisms, mentioned above and the infected cell must be destroyed. Antigen peptide-class I MHC is recognized by naïve CD8+ T cells, or precursor cytotoxic T cells (pCTL). Without Type 1 cytokine interleukin-2 (IL-2) produced by activated CD4+ Th1 cells, the naïve CD8+ T cell cannot differentiate to a mature CTL.

Natural killer cells destroy virally infected cells and tumors, but do not destroy cells infected with other infectious agents. The mode of recognition involves the presence of viral proteins on the infected cell membrane. Most infectious agents do not bud from the cell and leave their proteins exposed on the cell surface. Antibody-dependent cell-mediated cytotoxicity is the mechanism of natural killer cell recognition and killing that has been most extensively researched.

REVIEW OF KEY TERMS AND ABBREVIATIONS

Matching: Match the key term in the left column with the definition in the right column.

1. _____ MALT   a) this attaches to proteins targeted for degradation

2. _____ rubor   b) membrane attack complex on bacterial surface

3. _____ histamine   c) swelling

4. _____ inflammation   d) redness

5. _____ C3a and C5a

6. _____ IL-1 and TNF

7. _____ diapedesis

8. _____ Thp cells

9. _____ proteasome

10. _____ ubiquitin

11. _____ *Mycobacterium tuberculosis*

12. _____ edema

13. _____ osmotic lysis

14. _____ MHC

15. _____ CTL

16. _____ IgG

17. _____ IgM

18. _____ calor

19. _____ dolor

20. _____ anaphylatoxin

21. _____ interferon gamma

e) T helper precursor cells

f) causative agent of tuberculosis

g) cytotoxic T lymphocyte

h) heat

i) major histocompatibility complex

j) pain

k) activated B cells differentiate and secrete these

l) C5a induces mast cells/ basophils to degranulate

m) released in degranulation of mast cells, basophils

n) isotype switching to this secretion

o) anaphylatoxins and C3b crucial for immunity

p) large multimeric complex of several proteases

q) monocytes to macrophages; type 1 cytokine

r) neutrophils squeeze into infection site

s) tissue damage or infectious agents initiate this

t) mucosa associated lymphoid tissues

u) activated macrophages secrete these cytokines

Definitions: Write the definition of each of the following words or terms.

1. MALT _____

_____

2. histamine _____

_____

3. bradykinin _____

_____

4. osmotic lysis _____

_____

5. anaphylatoxins _____

_____

6. interleukin-1 and TNF _____

_____

7. chemotactic _____

_____

8. diapedesis _____

_____

9. Thp cells _____

_____

10. interferon gamma _____

_____

11. *Mycobacterium tuberculosis* _____

_____

12. proteasome _____

_____

13. ubiquitin _____

_____

REVIEW EXERCISES

True or False: Read each statement and decide if it is TRUE or FALSE. Place T or F on the line before each statement.

1. _____   CD4+ T cells can be activated when the infectious agent is in the cytosol of any cell in the body.

2. _____   Natural killer cells destroy bacterially infected cells.

3. _____   Microbes thriving in the phagosome are classified as intracellular organisms.

4. _____   Most infectious agents bud from the cell and leave their proteins exposed on the cell surface.

5. _____ Complexity of host defense mechanisms, and how they function to orchestrate an immune response, can be simplified by approaching host defense from the perspective of the location of the infectious agent.

Fill in the Blank: Complete the following sentences on the immune system by filling in the missing word or words.

1. There are only three locations for infectious agents—outside the cell, inside a(n) _____ , or inside the cytoplasm.

2. Neutrophils function in the process called _____ .

3. The vascular endothelium becomes more permeable so that circulating cells can get to the infected tissue because of _____ that is from degranulation of mast cells.

4. Antigen presentation to CD4+ T cells is the function of _____ .

5. _____ differentiate to antibody secreting plasma cells.

Multiple Choice: Choose the best answer.

1. How can a microbe become pathogenic and cause disease in a normal healthy individual?

   a. If the individual has been sick before.
   b. If the individual has been exposed to microbes.
   c. If microbes sabotage host defense components.
   d. If the microbes enter interstitial fluid.
   e. If the microbes are intracellular.

2. Degranulation of inflammatory mediators that include histamine is a function of

   a. tissue macrophages.
   b. CD4+ T cells.
   c. B cells.
   d. mast cells.
   e. neutrophils.

3. This anaphylatoxin binds to mast cells and basophils, inducing their degranulation, which results in the release of histamine.

   a. kallikrein
   b. bradykinin
   c. IL-1
   d. TNF
   e. C5a

4. The insertion of the membrane attack complex on the bacterial surface causes one of the following.

   a. complement activation
   b. degranulation
   c. osmotic lysis
   d. cascade
   e. chemotaxis

CRITICAL THINKING EXERCISE

Critical Thinking 1: Read this scenario and then answer the questions that follow.

Tom reads about interleukin-1 and tumor necrosis factor acting on the human body to induce fever. Sarah remembers effects of other immunological molecules, too. Tom wonders why fever is such a part of infection, but Sarah seems to remember an answer to that from her human anatomy and physiology.

1. What is the name of the class of molecules Tom is referring to with the IL-1 and TNF? (What part of the body do they act upon to cause elevated body temperature?)

2. What other molecules are there in the class of molecules Tom is referring to and what other effects might they have?

3. What answer does Sarah have from human anatomy and physiology for why fever is such a part of infection? (Tom has part of the answer from immunology, and then Sarah remembers something about the effect of elevated temperature, if *not* prolonged or excessive, on the human body and its processes.)

CASE STUDY

Some students you know are preparing a project for the immunology class on cells of the immune system that demonstrates phagocytosis. They outline the whole process of phagocytosis in these cells, showing many similarities in the function of the cells. Also, these students make it a point to cover how these cells get where they need to be to do the work they do for the immune system.

1. What do the students mention in their project about the function of phagocytosis? (How do the cells get where they need to be?)

2. What cells are the students talking about when they bring up this topic?

3. The students mention how similar the phagocytes are, but what makes them different? (Contrast these phagocytes by structure and function.)

Section II
LABORATORY TECHNIQUES

CHAPTER 10

INSTRUMENTATION

OUTLINE

- Instrumentation for Measurement of Antigen-Antibody Interactions
  - Gamma Ray Emission, Fluorescence, and Chemiluminescence
- Instrumentation for Measuring Color Intensity
  - Spectrophotometers and Photometers
- Instrumentation for Measuring Chemiluminescence
  - Luminometer
- Instrumentation for Measuring Fluorescence
  - Factors That Affect Fluorescence Measurements
  - Spectrofluorometers and Filter Fluorometers
  - Flow Cytometers
  - Fluorescence Microscope
- Instrumentation for Detecting Radioactivity
  - Radioactivity
  - Gamma Counter: Solid Scintillation Detector Counter
- Instrumentation for Detecting Non-Labeled Immune Complexes
  - Nephelometry
  - Turbidimetry

OBJECTIVES

Upon completion of this chapter, the reader should be able to:

1. Understand the basic principles of instruments that measure the intensity of colored solutions: spectrophotometer and photometer.
2. Understand the basic principles of chemiluminescence and the luminometer.
3. Understand the basic principles of fluorescence and the instruments that measure fluorescence: spectrofluorometer, fluorometer, fluorescence microscope, flow cytometry.
4. Understand the basic principles of radioactivity and the instruments that measure gamma radiation.
5. Understand the basic principles of nephelometry and turbidimetry as well as the instrumentation for detecting unlabeled immune complexes.

SUMMARY OF KEY POINTS

Instrumentation used to detect antigen-antibody interactions depends on whether or not an indicator label has been linked to an antibody or antigen molecule. The type of label dictates the instrumentation used to measure formation of antibody-antigen complexes.

Alkaline phosphatase is often used as an indicator molecule with immunoassays using enzymes linked to antibodies (antigen) in the system. Enzymes are indirect indicators dependent on their effect on the substrate to determine the type of response and the instrument needed for detection. Spectrophotometers or photometers may be used, for example, to determine the intensity of color and relative amount of antigen-antibody complex formed in situations in which the substrate becomes a colored product after enzymatic action. Ideally, intensity of color is directly proportional to the antigen-antibody complex formation. If there is a chemiluminescent intermediate, instrumentation used to detect antigen-antibody interaction is a luminometer. Ideally, emitted light intensity is directly proportional to the amount of chemiluminescent intermediate formed, which is in turn proportional to the amount of antibody/antigen complexes made.

Fluorochromes, substances absorbing light at one wavelength and then emitting light called fluorescence of a longer wavelength, are used as indicator molecules in some immunoassays as well. Ideally, emitted light intensity is directly proportional to amount of fluorochrome present in the sample. Some of the absorbed energy is quickly dissipated as heat or vibrational energy instead of fluorescence; therefore, the emitted light has less energy than the light absorbed by the fluorochrome. Factors affecting the amount of fluorescence that is measured are (1) light scattering in the solution, (2) quenching by the solvent, (3) concentration quenching, (4) cuvette fluorescence, and (5) temperature. Spectrofluorometers, filter fluorometers, flow cytometers, or fluorescent microscopes each with unique features may be used to detect fluorescence.

Radioactive isotopes are useful in diagnosis of various disorders using radioimmunoassays. These diagnostic tests are based on competitive binding of unlabeled antigen and radiolabeled antigen for binding sites available on a limited number of antibody molecules. Stable molecules have the number of protons in the nucleus equal to the number of electrons orbiting the nucleus, an optimal ratio of neutrons to protons, and the nucleus has a tendency to have an even number of protons and neutrons. Any atom deviating from the optimal proton/neutron ratio is unstable, and unstable atoms alter the ratio of protons and neutrons spontaneously through radioactive decay until there is a stable ration achieved. There is alpha decay, beta decay, or electron capture. In electron capture, gamma rays are released from the atom, and these gamma rays are commonly measured in radioimmunoassays by a scintillation detector. Commonly used radioisotopes in the clinical laboratory are iodine 125 and iodine 131.

Without an indicator label, immune complexes can be detected by measuring the effect of collimated light on the sample. Collimated light has four different effects when it hits a particle (immune complexes): it may be absorbed, transmitted, reflected, and some may be scattered. Nephelometry measures the amount of light scatter, and turbidimetry is the measure of amount of light absorbed by the immune complexes.

REVIEW OF KEY TERMS AND ABBREVIATIONS

Matching: Match the key term in the left column with the definition in the right column.

1. _____ fluorochrome

2. _____ photometer

3. _____ alkaline phosphatase

4. _____ monochromator

5. _____ PMT

6. _____ chemiluminescence

7. _____ luminometer

8. _____ calibration curve

9. _____ wavelength

10. _____ excitation spectrum

11. _____ immunoassays

12. _____ quenching

13. _____ flow cytometers

14. _____ direct labeling

15. _____ indirect labeling

16. _____ ELISA

17. _____ fluorescence microscopes

18. _____ VDRL

19. _____ end point analysis

20. _____ NINIA

21. _____ precipitation curve

a) enzyme commonly used as indicator

b) longer when less energy, shorter when more

c) secondary antibody label targeting antibodies

d) measures chemiluminescence

e) detect cell surface molecules that fluoresce

f) venereal diseases research laboratory

g) ensures patient's sample is appropriate dilution

h) nephelometric inhibition immunoassay

i) in these, fluorochromes conjugated to antibodies

j) used in quantitation or structural features

k) also called a spectrophotometer

l) enzyme linked immunosorbent assay

m) wave selector for spectrophotometer

n) sample incubated with antibody for 24 hours

o) graphic representation of precipitation

p) photomultiplier tube

q) label is on the antibody directly interacting

r) light emitted from a chemical reaction

s) decrease in fluorescent intensity

t) fluorochrome "fingerprint"

u) indicator fluoresces

Definitions: Write the definition of each of the following words or terms.

1. monochromator _____

_____

2. filter _____

_____

3. photomultiplier tube _____

_____

4. luminometer _____

_____

5. wavelength _____

_____

6. quenching _____

_____

7. flow cytometer _____

_____

8. AIDS _____

_____

9. direct labeling _____

_____

10. indirect labeling _____

_____

11. ELISA _____

_____

12. fluorescence microscopes _____

_____

13. VDRL _____

_____

REVIEW EXERCISES

True or False: Read each statement and decide if it is TRUE or FALSE. Place T or F on the line before each statement.

1. _____ Fluorescence microscopy is commonly used to confirm a positive screening test (venereal diseases research laboratory) for syphilis.

2. _____ When collimated light hits a particle (e.g., immune complexes) in solution, there are at least four effects: absorption, transmissions, reflection, and scattering.

3. _____ Nephelometers are instruments that measure the amount of radioactivity in a sample.

4. _____ Performance of light scattering assays do not depend on the quality of reagents.

5. _____ The generation of a colored product (by the action of an enzyme on a substrate) is measured with a spectrophotometer or photometer.

Fill in the Blank: Complete the following sentences on the immune system by filling in the missing word or words.

1. _____ are all phenomenon that occur when unstable molecules or electrons assume or revert to a more stable state.

2. The enzyme _____ is commonly used as the indicator molecule.

3. The main difference between the spectrophotometer and photometer is the type of _____ .

4. In a spectrophotometer, the wave selector is a _____ .

5. _____ is the name given to the light emitted from a chemical reaction.

Multiple Choice: Choose the best answer.

1. Commonly used detector in spectrophotometer is the

   a. photomultiplier tube.
   b. cathode.
   c. galvanometer.
   d. cell sorter.
   e. radioactive isotope.

2. Light emitted from a chemical reaction is

   a. fluorescence.
   b. gamma radiation.
   c. chemiluminescence.
   d. amplification.
   e. quenching.

3. Sophisticated instrument in which cells in a liquid suspension flow past a laser beam, one at a time.

   a. ELISA
   b. RIA
   c. VDRL
   d. nephelometer
   e. flow cytometer

4. All of these are phenomena occurring when unstable molecules or electrons assume or revert to a more stable state except for

   a. gamma ray emission.
   b. fluorescence.
   c. chemiluminescence.
   d. reflection.
   e. b and d

CRITICAL THINKING EXERCISE

Tom and Sarah are wondering about nephelometry, and its advantages and disadvantages. Kim does not know about nephelometry at all, but she understands spectrophotometers.

1. How do Tom and Sarah explain nephelometry to Kim? How would they distinguish it from spectrophotometry?

2. What advantages are there to nephelometry? What are the disadvantages?

3. What about quality control in nephelometry? How do you distinguish nephelometry from turbidimetry?

CHAPTER 11

INDICATOR LABELS

OUTLINE

- Indicator-Labeled Immunoassays
  - Radioactive Isotopes
  - Fluorochromes
  - Enzyme-Linked Approach
- Methods of Coupling Indicator Labels to Antigens or Antibodies
  - The Biotin-(Strep)avidin-Indicator Label System
- Standard Curves in Immunoassays
  - Serial Dilutions of Standards
  - Single Dilutions
- Principles of Immunoassays That Use Indicator Labels
  - Using Protein A in Immunoassays
  - Competitive Binding Immunoassays
  - Non Competitive Immunoassays
- Indicator-Labeled Immunoassays: Nomenclature
  - Enzyme-Linked Immunosorbent Assay (ELISA)
  - Chemiluminescent Immunoassay (CLIA)
  - Enzyme-Multiplied Immunoassay Technique (EMIT)
  - Fluorescent Polarization Immunoassay (FPIA)
  - Radioimmunoassays (RIA)

OBJECTIVES

Upon completion of this chapter, the reader should be able to:

1. Describe the role of indicator labels in immunoassays.

2. Explain how radioactive isotopes, fluorochromes, and enzymes are used in indicator labeled immunoassays.

3. Describe how the (strep)avidin-biotin system functions to couple indicator molecules to antigens or antibodies.

4. Explain how the same enzyme can be used in one immunoassay to produce an end point that is a colored product, while in another immunoassay the product is a chemiluminescent intermediate.

5. Understand the difference between fluorescence and chemiluminescence.

6. Describe the general procedure for dilutions for constructing a standard/calibration curve and the role of the standard curve in indicator labeled immunoassays.

7. Describe the general procedures for competitive immunoassays.

8. Describe the general procedures for non-competitive immunoassays.

9. Compare and contrast the indirect immunoassay and the antibody sandwich non-competitive immunoassays.

10. Compare and contrast the principles of indicator labeled immunoassays including CLIA, ELISA, EMIT, FPIA, IRMA, RIA.

SUMMARY OF KEY POINTS

Antigen/antibody reactions form the basis of immunoassays, and although precipitation and agglutination are used to monitor the formation of antigen/antibody complexes, the use of indicator labels on antigens or antibodies can enhance sensitivity of the assays. Three broad areas describe indicator labels: radioactive isotopes, fluorochromes, and enzymes. Covalent linkage, glutaraldehyde, or (strept) avidin-biotin systems are all different methods by which an indicator label may be coupled to antigen or antibody.

Enzyme use is becoming increasingly popular, and alkaline phosphatase and horseradish peroxidase are used in indicator labeled immunoassays. These enzymes are indirect, depending on a substrate before there is a change in some measurable parameter. Colored products or chemiluminescence are two of the manifestations of enzyme activity depending on the substrate. Fluorochromes are another type of indicator molecule that absorb light and become transiently excited. The excited molecule, assuming a more stable state of energy, emits light that is called fluorescence. The nature of the stimulus causing molecular excitation differentiates fluorescence from chemiluminescence. Radioactive isotopes are important in the clinical laboratory for diagnosis of various disorders using radioimmunoassays.

There are two indicator labeled immunoassays classified as either competitive (used to measure presence of antigen in biological fluids and called RIA, FPIA, EMIT, and with radioactive isotopes IRMA) and non-competitive (indirect immunoassay designed to detect antibody in the biological sample, and antibody sandwich approach designed to detect antigen).

Immunoassays provide numerical measures proportional to antigen/antibody complexes present in the sample, but for many clinical tests it is necessary to know the actual concentration of antigen or antibody in the biological sample. Conversion of the numerical measures that are obtained into concentration can be done by interpolating those measures on a standard curve. Standard or calibration curves must be performed under identical conditions as the patient's samples to become the reference from which numerical data obtained from the patient's sample can be converted into an actual concentration. Standard reagents are serially diluted to construct a standard curve, and with each dilution measured with a known concentration of other reagents used in the assay.

The indicator label used in the assay will always determine instrumentation used for detecting bound antibody as described in Chapter 10.

REVIEW OF KEY TERMS AND ABBREVIATIONS

Matching: Match the key term in the left column with the definition in the right column.

1. _____ indicator labels

2. _____ fluorescence

3. _____ glutaraldhyde

4. _____ biotinylated antibody

5. _____ serial dilution

6. _____ competitive

7. _____ protein A

8. _____ EMIT

9. _____ FPIA

10. _____ RIA

11. _____ IRMA

12. _____ antibody sandwich assay

13. _____ horseradish peroxidase

14. _____ alkaline phosphatase

15. _____ (strept)avidin

16. _____ gamma rays

a) biotin coupled to antibody

b) radiolabeled immunoassay

c) repetitive dilution of a sample by the same amount

d) radioactive isotopes emit these (e.g., iodine 125)

e) binds to Fc of IgG (from cell wall of bacterium)

f) enzyme as indirect indicator label; from plants

g) immunoradiometric assay

h) quantitation: radioactive, fluorochrome, enzymes

i) designed to detect antigen in bodily fluids

j) labeled and non-labeled antigen compete

k) enzymes can be linked to this with biotin

l) fluorochrome immunoassay

m) energy emitted as visible light

n) enzyme multiplied immunoassay

o) enzyme as indirect indicator label; many species

p) bifunctional reagent cross links two amino acids

Definitions: Write the definition of each of the following words or terms.

1. alkaline phosphatase _____

_____

2. fluorescence _____

_____

3. horseradish peroxidase _____

_____

4. glutaraldehyde _____

_____

5. biotinylated antibody _____

_____

6. standard curve _____

_____

7. serial dilution _____

_____

8. competitive assays _____

_____

9. non-competitive assays _____

_____

10. RIA _____

_____

11. FIA _____

_____

12. ELISA _____

_____

13. FPIA _____

_____

REVIEW EXERCISES

True or False: Read each statement and decide if it is TRUE or FALSE. Place T or F on the line before each statement.

1. _____ Plane polarized light is electromagnetic radiation vibrating in only one direction rather than being scattered in all directions

2. _____ ELISA is a non-classical competitive immunoassay used for the detection of illegal and therapeutic drugs.

3. _____ Fluorochromes are catalysts for chemical reactions.

4. _____ Alkaline phosphatase is an enzyme commonly used as direct indicator labels.

5. _____ Glutaraldehyde is a bifunctional reagent covalently cross-linking two amino acids together.

Fill in the Blank: Complete the following sentences on the immune system by filling in the missing word or words.

1. Enzymes can be linked to _____ for use in systems in which biotin has been attached to either antigen or antibody.

2. As the excited molecule returns to a more stable state most of the energy is emitted as visible light that is called _____ .

3. Intensity of colored product can be determined using a _____ or a microtiter plate reader.

4. To convert numerical measures obtained into concentration, it is necessary to interpolate measurements onto a _____ .

5. _____ is the repetitive dilution of a sample by the same amount.

Multiple Choice: Choose the best answer.

1. Radioisotopes are used as labels; assay used to detect antigen in sample.

    a. RIA
    b. FIA
    c. FPIA
    d. EMIT
    e. ELISA

2. Indirect immunoassay approach is often referred to as this because there are three layers of reagents: antibody, antigen, and labeled secondary antibody.

    a. antigen-antibody complex technique
    b. sandwich technique
    c. IRMA technique
    d. EMIT technique
    e. RIA technique

3. This procedure is typically performed on urine samples, however, serum may be used.

   a. ELISA
   b. EMIT
   c. RIA
   d. FPIA
   e. IRMA

4. For competitive immunoassays, the indicator label is either

   a. radioisotope or horseradish peroxidase.
   b. alkaline phosphatase or fluorochrome.
   c. radioisotope or fluorochrome.
   d. antigen-X or anti-X antibodies.
   e. protein A or avidin.

CRITICAL THINKING EXERCISE

One of your friends is going to have a test to measure a certain hormone's level, and she thinks the test, as she understands it, has "something" to do with immunological techniques. Your friend realizes that you're taking immunology, so she comes to you.

1. What sort of immunoassay do you think that your friend is going to have?

2. How do you explain the procedure to your friend?

3. How many immunoassays are there in this category?

CASE STUDY

Someone in the nursing class has asked you to explain non-competitive immunoassays for their class tomorrow morning.

1. How do you describe these immunoassays to the nursing class?

2. Describe the protocols for these assays.

CHAPTER 12

PRECIPITATION

OUTLINE

OBJECTIVES

Upon completion of this chapter, the reader should be able to:

1. List the types of intermolecular interactions between antigen and antibody.
2. Explain the difference between affinity and avidity.
3. Describe the formation of antigen/antibody complexes and the lattice theory.
4. Compare and contrast the three zones that comprise a precipitation curve.
5. Explain the difference between single immunodiffusion and double immunodiffusion.
6. Describe the difference between single linear and radial immunodiffusion.
7. Describe the difference between double linear and double angular immunodiffusion.
8. Describe the three patterns that may arise in double angular immunodiffusion and provide a rationale for each of the three patterns observed.
9. Explain how rocket immunoelectrophoresis differs from radial immunodiffusion.
10. Explain how counter immunoelectrophoresis differs from double immunodiffusion.

SUMMARY OF KEY POINTS

Primary antigen/antibody interactions are the initial reactions between an antigen and an antibody, and these reactions are the result of non-covalent, intermolecular forces between the antigen and the Fab region of an antibody. Intermolecular forces include hydrogen bonds, ionic bonds, and van der Waals forces. Antibody affinity refers to the bond strength between the epitope and the region of the antibody with which it interacts within the Fab region. Avidity is the overall strength of the antigen/antibody interactions.

Secondary antigen/antibody reactions are those that occur following primary antigen/antibody interactions, and precipitation of the antigen/antibody complexes known as immunoprecipitation is an example. Conditions for immunoprecipitation are: the antigen must be multivalent and soluble, each antibody must have at least two available antigen binding sites, and the antigen and antibody must be present in correct proportions.

Precipitin curves are graphic representations of precipitin reactions occurring under specific experimental conditions, in which the concentration of one reactant is constant although the concentration of the second reagent is increased serially in test samples. Maximal precipitation occurs when each antigen and antibody molecule is cross-linked, and the point at which maximal precipitation occurs is called the zone of equivalence. Beyond the equivalence point in the experimental precipitation reaction, the addition of more antigen decreases the amount of precipitation formed until no precipitation is observed.

Immunoprecipitation may be used with a diffusion system, and the combined effect is called immunodiffusion. These systems are single linear diffusion, single radial diffusion, double simple immunodiffusion, and double angular immunodiffusion. The primary goal in immunodiffusion systems is to detect antigen/antibody interactions using precipitation as a measure of the reaction. Temperature, pH, and buffer type all contribute as factors in immunodiffusion, but the most important factor is the relative concentration of antigen and antibody. Single immunodiffusion systems are those in which one of the reactants (antigen or antibody) remains fixed in the gel and the other is allowed to move and interact with the immobilized reagent. They may be linear or radial. An applied voltage may be applied to modify the single immunodiffusion technique, and as a result the precipitation pattern assumes a rocket shape rather than a ring shape. Therefore, this voltage-mediated variation of single immunodiffusion is called rocket immunoelectrophoresis.

Double immunodiffusion systems are those in which both reactants are free to move, interact, and form complexes and precipitate when equivalence occurs. Single and angular are two techniques using classic double immunodiffusion, in which single has two parallel wells in the gel and reagents diffuse radially, and angular has three wells cut out of an agar gel and the three proteins diffuse in all directions. Patterns of precipitation differ in angular immunodiffusion depending on the relationship between the antigens in the two wells, and the antibody in the third well. Three patterns develop and are referred to as patterns of identity, partial identity, or non-identity.

REVIEW OF KEY TERMS AND ABBREVIATIONS

Matching: Match the key term in the left column with the definition in the right column.

1. _____ primary interactions	a)	based on diffusion of three reagents within agar
2. _____ electrostatic interactions	b)	antigens in 2 wells identical/specific for antibody
3. _____ affinity	c)	precipitation of antibody/antigen in lattice
4. _____ multivalent antigens	d)	between two oppositely charged ionic groups
5. _____ immunoprecipitation	e)	interactions between electron clouds
6. _____ univalent antigen	f)	precipitin pattern is radial
7. _____ flocculation	g)	maximal possible precipitant forms
8. _____ precipitin curve	h)	later part of the precipitin curve
9. _____ equivalence point	i)	antigens/antibodies are reagents; one fixed in gel
10. _____ zone of antibody excess	j)	applied voltage pushes antigen in gel with antibody
11. _____ immunodiffusion	k)	hydrogen and ionic bonds, Van der Waals forces
12. _____ Ouchterlony method	l)	precipitin reactions graphically represented
13. _____ zone of antigen excess	m)	voltage facilitated double immunodiffusion
14. _____ single linear	n)	have more than one epitope
15. _____ single radial	o)	hydrogen atom attracted to O or N
16. _____ rocket electrophoresis	p)	with one epitope
17. _____ counter electrophoresis	q)	early part of precipitin curve
18. _____ pattern of identity	r)	are also called ionic bonds
19. _____ hydrogen bond	s)	natural clumping

20. _____   ionic bond

t) diffusion of antigen and/or antibodies

21. _____   Van der Waals forces

u) refers to bond strength between epitope and Fab

Definitions: Write the definition of each of the following words or terms.

1. hydrogen bonds _____

_____

2. ionic bonds _____

_____

3. Van der Waals forces _____

_____

4. affinity _____

_____

5. avidity _____

_____

6. precipitation _____

_____

7. multivalent antigens _____

_____

8. univalent antigens _____

_____

9. flocculation _____

_____

10. precipitin curve _____

_____

11. equivalence point _____

_____

12. immunodiffusion _____

_____

REVIEW EXERCISES

True or False: Read each statement and decide if it is TRUE or FALSE. Place T or F on the line before each statement.

1. _____   Van der Waals forces are also referred to as electrostatic interactions.

2. _____   Overall association interaction between antibody and antigen is referred to as affinity.

3. _____   All monovalent antibodies have two Fab regions, pentameric antibodies like IgM have ten.

4. _____   Multi-determinant epitopes are different on the antigen.

5. _____   Cross-linking of antibodies occurs when the antigen is univalent.

Fill in the Blank: Complete the following sentences on the immune system by filling in the missing word or words.

1. _____ of antibodies occurs only when the antigen is multivalent.

2. _____ structure occurs when one antigen molecule cross-links more than one antibody.

3. Precipitation of antigen/antibody complexes is often referred to as _____ .

4. _____ is a graphic representation of precipitin reactions occurring under specific experimental conditions.

5. The size of precipitant increases as the antigen concentration is increased until the maximal possible precipitant forms, which is referred to as the _____ .

Multiple Choice: Choose the best answer.

1. Observed when a suspension of antigens and antibodies is agitated.

   a. lattice formation
   b. precipitation
   c. flocculation
   d. equivalence point
   e. immunodiffusion

2. Phenomenon referring to the diffusion of antigen and/or antibodies.

   a. lattice formation
   b. precipitation
   c. flocculation
   d. equivalence point
   e. immunodiffusion

3. Applied voltage pushes antigen through an antibody containing gel.

   a. single immunodiffusion
   b. radial immunodiffusion
   c. double immunodiffusion
   d. rocket immunoelectrophoresis
   e. Ouchterlony method

4. Three reagents diffusing in all directions within agar or agarose in a petri dish.

   a. double simple immunodiffusion
   b. counter immunoelectrophoresis
   c. rocket immunoelectrophoresis
   d. Ouchterlony method
   e. immunodiffusion

CRITICAL THINKING EXERCISE

Tom is complaining to Sarah that just when he had figured out a lot about immunology, he had to know more chemistry and physics than he had previously thought. After Sarah stops laughing, she asks him why he thinks that, to which Tom replies that Chapter 12 refers to antibody/antigen interactions he didn't understand in chemistry and physics, but now they turn up in immunology class.

1. What do you think Tom is talking about? And, why?

2. What could Sarah say to help Tom with this information.

3. Describe the phenomena for primary and secondary antigen/antibody reactions necessary for Tom to learn now.

CASE STUDY

Tom's uncle is going to have some testing done in a medical laboratory. All Tom can get out of his uncle is that the test will measure apoproteins. Tom knows that his uncle is worried about his cholesterol and triglyceride levels, and he has started a new diet along with a new exercise routine. Tom's uncle has been on a statin type medication.

1. From Chapter 12, what has Tom learned about apoproteins and how they might be measured?

2. Describe the test and what techniques are used in its implementation.

3. What is a statin? What sort of diet might Tom's uncle be on?

CHAPTER 13

ELECTROPHORESIS

OUTLINE

OBJECTIVES

Upon completion of this chapter, the reader should be able to:

1. Explain the principle of protein separation using electrophoresis.
2. Understand the role of pH in the electrophoretic separation of proteins.
3. Explain endo-osmosis and its effect on the migration of proteins.
4. List the various non-soluble supports for electrophoresis as well as the advantages and disadvantages of each.
5. Describe the basic principles and general protocols for (a) classic immunoelectrophoresis, (b) immunofixation, (c) rocket immunoelectrophoresis, (d) counter immunoelectrophoresis, (e) crossed immunoelectrophoresis, and (f) zone electrophoresis.

SUMMARY OF KEY POINTS

Electrophoresis is a technique in which charged molecules are separated when an electric field is applied to the system via oppositely charged electrodes, termed cathode (negatively charged) and anode (positively charged); so, particles that are negatively charged move toward the anode, and those positively charged move toward the cathode. The rate at which a molecule will migrate in the presence of this applied electric field is influenced by the charge of the molecule, its size and shape, pH of the buffer, and the strength of the electric field. Proteins are charged molecules and will not migrate if the pH of the buffer is such that the positive charges on the protein balance the negative charges. The isoelectric point for a given protein (pI) is the pH at which a protein is neutral, and when the pH equals the pI, the molecule will not migrate under the influence of an electric field.

Support media used for electrophoresis include filter paper, cellulose acetate, polyacrylamide gel, and agarose gel. Some support media have charged groups on their surface and this can lead to a problem known as endo-osmosis or electro-osmosis. Ions in the buffer bind to the charged groups, causing this problem.

Prior introduction of specific antibodies into the gel and the observation of a precipitin band can detect electrophoretically separated proteins. This precipitin band forms when the serum protein of interest (antigen) binds to the antibodies at concentrations forming the zone of equivalence. Classically, serum proteins are first separated by electrophoresis, then antibody is introduced in a trough located parallel to the separated proteins. Antigen and antibody diffuse toward one another without the influence of the electric field. Where they meet, a characteristic precipitin arc is observed. In immunofixation after electrophoresis of serum proteins, antibodies are introduced into the gel by application on the surface of each electrophoretic track. In crossed immunoelectrophoresis, the proteins are first electrophoretically separated in one direction, are then an electric field is applied from a different angle.

In some techniques, the electrophoretic separation of proteins and the antigen/antibody interaction occurs all in one step. Rocket immunoelectrophoresis forces antigen through an antibody containing gel. A rocket shape precipitin pattern is thus produced. In counter-immunoelectrophoresis, antigen and antibody are placed in opposite sides of the gel, but in line with one another.

SDS-PAGE is an electrophoretic technique in which proteins are first pretreated with sodium dodecyl sulphate (SDS), which is a negatively charged denaturing agent. SDS-treated proteins have an overall negative charge and so separation is based on molecular weight, not charge.

REVIEW OF KEY TERMS AND ABBREVIATIONS

Matching: Match the key term in the left column with the definition in the right column.

1. _____ electrophoresis

2. _____ cathode

3. _____ anode

4. _____ non-soluble media

5. _____ isoelectric point

6. _____ denature

7. _____ endo-osmosis

8. _____ agar

9. _____ agarose

10. _____ cellulose acetate

11. _____ polyacrylamide gels

12. _____ densitometer

13. _____ 2D-IEF

14. _____ immunofixation

15. _____ Laurell Technique

16. _____ SDS-PAGE

a) constrain molecule movements; used for separation

b) linear polysaccharide component of agar

c) net flow of hydrated ions in one direction in electric field

d) rocket immunoelectrophoresis

e) cellulose with acetic anhydride; support medium

f) pass a light beam through stained cellulose acetate strip

g) negatively charged electrode

h) SDS (detergent) polyacrylamide gel electrophoresis

i) two dimensional immunoelectrophoresis

j) pH unique for each protein in which charges balance

k) proteins unfold; shape is altered

l) technique: molecules separated by charge in electric field

m) protein separation followed by immunoprecipitation

n) polysaccharide mixture of agarose and agaropectin

o) polymerized acrylamide cross-linked with reagent

p) positively charged electrode

Definitions: Write the definition of each of the following words or terms.

1. electrophoresis _____

   _____

2. non-soluble support media _____

   _____

3. isoelectric point _____

   _____

4. electro-osmosis _____

   _____

5. agar _____

   _____

6. agarose _____

   _____

7. cellulose acetate _____

   _____

8. zone electrophoresis _____

   _____

9. classic immunoelectrophoresis _____

   _____

10. crossed immunoelectrophoresis _____

   _____

11. immunofixation _____

   _____

12. counter immunoelectrophoresis _____

   _____

13. rocket immunoelectrophoresis _____

   _____

REVIEW EXERCISES

True or False: Read each statement and decide if it is TRUE or FALSE. Place T or F on the line before each statement.

1. _____ The cathode is the positively charged electrode.

2. _____ Soluble support media constrain molecule movement and so are used for the separation of biological molecules.

3. _____ Electrophoresis is useful for the separation of proteins present in serum, urine, and cerebrospinal fluid.

4. _____ The isoelectric point is the certain pH in which the positive charges on the protein balance the negative charges

5. _____ High temperatures cause proteins to unfold (denature).

Fill in the Blank: Complete the following sentences on the immune system by filling in the missing word or words.

1. _____ is a term used to refer to the net flow of hydrated ions in one direction in which the electric field is applied.

2. _____ is a polysaccharide mixture of agarose and agaropectin.

3. _____ is prepared by treating cellulose with acetic anhydride.

4. _____ is a technique in which proteins or nucleic acids are separated and localize into separate bands or zones.

5. Proteins are not visible on the cellulose acetate, so they are histochemically stained for protein and then scanned using a _____ .

Multiple Choice: Choose the best answer.

1. Used to identify antigens on bacteria, fungi, or viruses present in biological fluids (e.g., hepatitis B antigen). (agar gel)

   a. counter electrophoresis
   b. classic immunoelectrophoresis
   c. immunofixation electrophoresis
   d. rocket immunoelectrophoresis
   e. crossed immunoelectrophoresis

2. Very time consuming; used to detect subtle differences in protein. (agarose)

   a. counter electrophoresis
   b. classic immunoelectrophoresis
   c. immunofixation electrophoresis
   d. rocket immunoelectrophoresis
   e. crossed immunoelectrophoresis

3. Quantitation of antigen specific for antibody in gel. Tests Factor VIII related antigens. (agarose gel)

    a. counter immunoelectrophoresis
    b. classic immunoelectrophoresis
    c. immunofixation electrophoresis
    d. rocket immunoelectrophoresis
    e. crossed immunoelectrophoresis

4. Primarily used for detection, or monitoring, myeloma proteins. Fast and sensitive system in agarose gel.

    a. classic immunoelectrophoresis
    b. crossed immunoelectrophoresis
    c. immunofixation electrophoresis
    d. rocket immunoelectrophoresis
    e. counter immunoelectrophoresis

CRITICAL THINKING EXERCISE

While talking to a nurse who has recently returned from Africa, you find out that immunological tests were used for diagnosis in certain hospitals. This doesn't surprise you, but the fact that some of the tests were electrophoresis-based does.

1. What is electrophoresis, and how might it be useful in a medical situation?

2. What sorts of electrophoretic tests could be useful in diagnosis?

3. Describe the tests and what disorders they might diagnose. Why were you surprised that electrophoresis was used?

CHAPTER 14

AGGLUTINATION

OUTLINE

- Agglutination
- Principles of Agglutination
  - Determining Antibody Titer
  - Factors That Affect Agglutination
- Agglutination Techniques
  - Slide Tests
  - Microtiter Plate Tests
- Types of Agglutination Reactions
  - Direct Agglutination
  - Indirect Agglutination
  - Reverse Agglutination
  - Latex Particle Agglutination Inhibition Reaction
  - Quantitative Agglutination Reactions
  - Hemagglutination
  - Viral Hemagglutination/Nonimmune Agglutination
  - Viral Hemagglutination Inhibition
- Antiglobulins Tests
  - Direct Coombs' Test
  - Indirect Coombs' Agglutination Test
- Applications of the Agglutination/Hemagglutination Reaction
  - Determination of ABO Blood Groups
  - Cold Autoagglutinins

- Febrile Agglutinins
- Heterophile Agglutination
- Autoimmune Disorders

OBJECTIVES

Upon completion of this chapter, the reader should be able to:

1. Explain the principles of the agglutination reaction and list the factors that affect the reaction.
2. Describe how antibody titer is determined and reported.
3. Explain why the agglutination reaction is a popular screening test for many infectious diseases.
4. Describe the basic principles and general protocols for the following tests: (a) direct agglutination, (b) indirect agglutination, (c) reverse agglutination, (d) latex agglutination inhibition, and (e) hemagglutination.
5. Explain why viral hemagglutination is classed as non-immune agglutination.
6. Describe the basic principles and general protocol for the viral agglutination test.
7. Compare and contrast hemagglutination, the direct Coombs' test, and the indirect Coombs' test.
8. List several applications of the agglutination test and describe the relevant antigen/antibody interactions on which the test is based.

SUMMARY OF KEY POINTS

Clumping and sedimentation of particulate antigen/antibody complexes is agglutination. It is used for visual detection of antigen/antibody reactions in diagnostic clinical tests for both infectious and non-infectious diseases. Agglutination tests may be performed using undiluted or diluted serum. Undiluted sera or 1:20 dilution are used for screening tests. After a positive screening test, samples are then serially diluted and retested using either tubes or a microtiter plate to ascertain the antibody titer. The antibody titer is reported as the reciprocal of that dilution beyond which no agglutination is seen. The equivalence zone is that appropriate relative concentration of antigen and antibody in which cross-linking and lattice formation occurs.

Several factors affect agglutination including buffer pH, relative concentration of antibody and antigen, location and concentration of antigenic determinants on the particle, electrostatic interactions between particles, electrolyte concentration, antibody isotype, and temperature. Agglutination is a useful screening test to determine if a patient has developed antibodies specific for an antigen. Techniques for agglutination may be done using slides, test tubes, or microtiter plates. Slides are used for screening large numbers of sera, while the tube or microtiter plate tests are used to confirm positive results from a slide test.

Agglutination reactions may be referred to as direct (active) or indirect (passive) depending on whether the antigen is intrinsic to the particle or has been absorbed or reacted with the particle. Agglutination tests to measure antigen concentration, rather than antibody, are reverse agglutination assay and agglutination inhibition reaction.

When red blood cells are agglutinated either by direct agglutination or indirect techniques, the technique is called hemagglutination. In direct hemagglutination, the antigen is an integral part of the red blood cell (the ABO blood group antigens), while in the indirect method soluble antigens (thyroglobulin, viral antigens) are complexed with red blood cells. Red blood cells are negatively charged as a result of sialic acid residues on their cell surface, and this is a problem associated with red blood cells in hemagglutination reactions. An electrostatic potential called the zeta potential is generated around the red blood cell when it is in solution; which does not impede the agglutination of IgM, but does impede IgG because the red blood cells repel one another and do not come close enough to allow for cross-linking. Coombs' reagent overcomes this problem crosslinking IgG molecules bound to the red blood cell.

Viruses have non-serological hemagglutinating properties, which means they can agglutinate red blood cells without any antibody. Viral hemagglutinin inhibition assay is used to detect viral antibodies in biological fluid (serum). When the infectious agent is not available in a biological fluid, a measurement of the anti-viral antibodies can provide diagnostic information

Commercially available tests use latex particles coated with antigen (or antibody) of interest. Any soluble antigen or antibody that can be affixed to the latex particle can then be used for an agglutination test. Tests are available for numerous infectious agents.

REVIEW OF KEY TERMS AND ABBREVIATIONS

Matching: Match the key term in the left column with the definition in the right column.

1. ____	ABO blood group	a) agglutination of red blood cells
2. ____	agglutination	b) fluid is tested for antigens; antibody is part of particle
3. ____	agglutinin	c) reported as reciprocal of dilution under consideration
4. ____	agglutinogen	d) protein secreted into blood in inflammatory response
5. ____	antibody titer	e) disperse dye immunoassay
6. ____	Coombs' reagent	f) visible clumping/sedimentation of antigen/antibody
7. ____	C-reactive protein	g) red blood cells in solution generate electrostatic potential
8. ____	hemagglutination	h) serum very dilute shows little or no agglutination
9. ____	HCG	i) large immune complexes form by antibody interactions
10. ____	IMPACT	j) human chorionic gonadotrophin
11. ____	postzone phenomenon	k) associated antigens, which interact with antibody
12. ____	prozone phenomenon	l) antigens intrinsic to red blood cells

13. _____ reverse agglutination

    m) anti-human IgG antibody binds to human Fcγ region

14. _____ SPIA

    n) serum very positive and undiluted shows no agglutination

15. _____ Todd units

    o) highest dilution resulting in agglutination

16. _____ zeta potential

    p) assays in which colloidal particle is inorganic

17. _____ DIA

    q) antibodies that agglutinate antigen

18. _____ lattices

    r) immunoassay by particle counting

Definitions: Write the definition of each of the following words or terms.

1. agglutination _____

   _____

2. lattice formation _____

   _____

3. antibody titer _____

   _____

4. zone of equivalence _____

   _____

5. electrolytes _____

   _____

6. slide test _____

   _____

7. microtiter plates _____

   _____

8. direct agglutination _____

   _____

9. indirect agglutination _____

   _____

10. HCG _____

_____

11. sol particle immunoassays _____

_____

12. disperse dye immunoassay _____

_____

13. zeta potential _____

_____

REVIEW EXERCISES

True or False: Read each statement and decide if it is TRUE or FALSE. Place T or F on the line before each statement.

1. _____ Agglutination is the clumping and sedimentation of particulate antigen/antibody complexes.

2. _____ Precipitation reactions involve particulate antigens while agglutination involves soluble antigens.

3. _____ Antibody titer is the highest dilution of the biological sample resulting in agglutination with no agglutination at any higher dilution.

4. _____ The slide test is used primarily for screening large numbers of sera.

5. _____ In direct agglutination, the antigen is an intrinsic component of the particle (e.g., bacterium).

Fill in the Blank: Complete the following sentences on the immune system by filling in the missing word or words.

1. Antibodies that agglutinate antigen are referred to as _____ .

2. _____ are large immune complexes that form as a result of antibody interactions with multivalent antigens.

3. _____ is the highest dilution of the biological sample still resulting in agglutination, with no agglutination being observed at higher dilutions.

4. The region between prozone and post zone phenomena in which maximal agglutination occurs is called the _____ .

5. _____ play a role in agglutination in that they reduce electrostatic charges that interfere with lattice formation.

Multiple Choice: Choose the best answer.

1. Clumping and sedimentation of particulate antigen/antibody complexes.

    a. agglutinogens
    b. flocculation
    c. agglutination
    d. precipitation
    e. lattices

2. Highest dilution of biological samples still resulting in agglutination.

    a. antigen titer
    b. antibody titer
    c. zone phenomena
    d. zone of equivalence
    e. post zone phenomenon

3. Serum samples that are strongly positive and undiluted show little or no agglutination.

    a. prozone phenomenon
    b. post zone phenomenon
    c. zone of equivalence
    d. precipitation
    e. lattice

4. All are factors affecting agglutination *except*

    a. buffer pH.
    b. antibody isotype.
    c. temperature.
    d. electrostatic interactions between particles.
    e. all of the above are factors.

CRITICAL THINKING EXERCISE

Tom, Sarah, and Kim are discussing agglutination before class one day. Tom wants to know what it is exactly, while Sarah is unsure of all the factors involved. Kim is most interested in the sorts of immunological tests using agglutination.

1. How would you define agglutination to Tom so he is ready for class?

2. What factors affect agglutination? Discuss them so Sarah will be prepared.

3. What immunological tests use agglutination?

CHAPTER 15

MOLECULAR DIAGNOSTIC TECHNOLOGY

OUTLINE

- Molecular Diagnostic Technology
- Nucleic Acids
  - Deoxyribonucleic Acid
  - Ribonucleic Acids
- Molecular Biology Tools
  - Restriction Endonucleases
  - Primers and Probes
  - Complementary DNA
- Amplification of Nucleic Acids
  - Polymerase Chain Reaction
  - Reverse Transcribed Polymerase Chain Reaction
  - Nucleic Acid Sequence Based Amplification
  - Transcription Mediated Amplification
  - Second Generation Nucleic Acid Amplification Strategies
- Signal Amplification Assays
  - Branched DNA
  - Hybrid Capture System
- Capture and Detection Techniques
  - Amplicons
  - Signal Amplification Assays
- Molecular Blotting Techniques

■ Southern Blot
■ Northern Blot
■ Western Blot
■ Detecting Genetic Mutations in Clinical Laboratories
■ Sickle Cell Disease: RFLP and Southern Blotting
■ Fragile X Syndrome: PCR and Southern Blotting

OBJECTIVES

Upon completion of this chapter, the reader should be able to:

1. Describe the building blocks of DNA and RNA.
2. Compare and contrast the structure and building blocks of DNA and RNA.
3. Understand the role of DNA polymerase in DNA replication.
4. Explain the role of transcription and translation in the synthesis of proteins.
5. Describe the role of restriction nucleases in bacteria and in molecular biology.
6. Explain the role of oligonucleotides in molecular biology techniques including the polymerase chain reaction and southern blotting.
7. Describe one cycle of the polymerase chain reaction and explain the rationale for varying the temperature during the cycle.
8. Explain the term restriction fragment length polymorphism and how RFLP plays a role in the clinical laboratory.
9. Compare and contrast molecular diagnostic tests based on nucleic acid amplification.
10. Compare and contrast molecular diagnostic tests based on signal amplification.
11. Compare and contrast the southern blot, northern blot, and western blot techniques.
12. Describe the role of PCR, southern blotting, and western blotting in the clinical laboratory.

SUMMARY OF KEY POINTS

Molecular biology tests, in which specific sequences of DNA or RNA are targeted for analysis, represent the most recent developments in clinical laboratory tests. They are used for diagnosis of genetic diseases, malignancies, tissue typing, paternity determination, and detection of infectious agents in biological samples.

Restriction nucleases (restriction enzymes or restriction endonucleases) are bacterial proteins, which cleave phage (viral) DNA as a bacterial defense, but these restriction nucleases can be used to cleave any DNA expressing the sequence recognized by the enzyme. DNA fragments left from these enzymes are called restriction fragments, and analysis of these fragments is called restriction fragment length polymorphism (RFLP). Restriction fragments are separated on a gel and analyzed by southern blotting, which requires that an oligonucleotide probe complementary to the DNA of interest be available. This test is used to identify carriers of sickle cell gene, as RFLP can be used to identify certain mutations in some diseases when the mutation occurs at a site normally cleaved by a restriction enzyme. RFLP is also used for fragile X syndrome for genetic counseling. Another technique known as western blotting is used to clinically detect antibodies specific to proteins present on a nitrocellulose or nylon membrane. Immune complexes are identified by labeled antibodies when the patient's antibodies are specific for the membrane-immobilized proteins. The diagnosis of Lyme disease and confirmatory test for infection with HIV are both done by western blotting techniques.

Polymerase chain reaction is a technique in which specific segments of DNA are amplified for analysis. Primers target the DNA adjacent to the DNA of interest, and then DNA is initiated for replication by polymerases.

Nucleic amplification techniques involve a sequence of DNA or RNA amplified, while signal amplification is where a number of indicator labels that target a nucleic acid hybrid is increased greatly. With signal amplification, hybrids can be detected even when they are few in number. Nucleic acids amplified are called amplicons, regardless of whether the product is DNA or RNA. Labeled probes able to hybridize to the product or target sequence are required to detect nucleic acids, and the commonly used probes are similar to those used for antibody detection in ELISA assays (alkaline phosphatase, biotin, horseradish peroxidase). Acridium ester and ruthenium are other types of labels. Instrumentation used for detection depends on the indicator label.

REVIEW OF KEY TERMS AND ABBREVIATIONS

Matching: Match the key term in the left column with the definition in the right column.

1. _____ acridium ester

2. _____ adenine

3. _____ amino acid

4. _____ amplicon

5. _____ plasmids

6. _____ autoradiography

7. _____ base pair

8. _____ branched DNA

9. _____ codon

10. _____ complementary

11. _____ cDNA

12. _____ cytosine

13. _____ DNA

14. _____ deoxynucleotides

a) branches of DNA bind lots of indicator labels

b) G is said to be this to C

c) made of two chains interacting by hydrogen bonds

d) triplet of bases encoding each amino acid

e) sugar in DNA

f) related to southern blotting, technique used to reveal location of radioactivity

g) excess labeled probes in hybridization protection assay

h) DNA is a polymer of these four different units

i) pyrimidine base that pairs with guanine

j) genomic DNA

k) building blocks for proteins

l) like southern, only RNA, not DNA, is extracted

m) adenine with thymine, cytosine with guanine

n) replication of DNA requires these special enzymes

15. _____ deoxyribose

16. _____ DNA polymerases

17. _____ double helix

18. _____ ethidium bromide

19. _____ gDNA

20. _____ hybrid

21. _____ northern blot

o) circular, extrachromosomal genetic material

p) dye intercalates in DNA and fluoresces in UV

q) from RNA template using reverse transcriptase

r) interaction of 2 complementary strands of nucleic acids

s) purine base always pairs with thymine

t) encodes genetic information for life

u) amplified nucleic acids

Definitions: Write the definition of each of the following words or terms.

1. annealing _____

_____

2. western blot _____

_____

3. fragile X syndrome _____

_____

4. sickle cell disease _____

_____

5. methylation _____

_____

6. southern blot _____

_____

7. nucleic acids _____

_____

8. ribose _____

_____

9. uracil _____

_____

10. hnRNA _____

_____

11. transcription _____

_____

12. processing (splicing) _____

_____

13. translation _____

_____

REVIEW EXERCISES

True or False: Read each statement and decide if it is TRUE or FALSE. Place T or F on the line before each statement.

1. _____ The sugar molecules are covalently linked via phosphodiester bonds in the deoxyribonucleotides.

2. _____ G is complementary to T, and C is complementary to A in DNA.

3. _____ Primers of about five nucleic acids are not necessary for replication.

4. _____ RNA is a single stranded molecule made up of four building blocks called ribonucleotides.

5. _____ In RNA uracil pairs with thymine.

Fill in the Blank: Complete the following sentences on the immune system by filling in the missing word or words.

1. Molecular diagnostic tests are those in which specific sequences of _____ is/are targeted for analysis.

2. _____ are macromolecules found in all living cells.

3. Four different _____ make up the chains covalently linked in the DNA linear polymer.

4. Watson and Crick described DNA as a _____ .

5. Base interactions (A, T, C, G) in the double stranded DNA are always adenine with thymine, while guanine always pairs with cytosine; this is called _____ .

Multiple Choice: Choose the best answer.

1. In DNA adenine always pairs with

   a. cytosine.
   b. guanine.
   c. uracil.
   d. thymine.
   e. thymidine.

2. When a cell divides, the entire DNA content is

   a. transcribed.
   b. translated.
   c. templated.
   d. complementary base paired.
   e. replicated.

3. In RNA uracil pairs with

   a. adenine.
   b. thymine.
   c. cytosine.
   d. guanine.
   e. thymidine.

4. Interaction of two complementary strands of nucleic acids is referred to as

   a. translation.
   b. transcription.
   c. duplication.
   d. replication.
   e. hybridization.

CRITICAL THINKING EXERCISE

Tom doesn't understand complementary base pairing because when he committed it to memory for DNA, he realized some other pairing was evident with RNA. Sarah tells him that he just needs to get some things straight about nucleic acids and their composition.

1. What probably got Tom confused about base pairing?

2. What does Sarah mean by her comment that Tom "just needs to get some things straight about nucleic acids and their composition"?

3. Contrast and compare DNA with RNA.

CASE STUDY

Your class went on a field trip to a clinical laboratory. While there, the technician mentioned the use of restriction enzymes and how very important they were for their work.

1. What are restriction enzymes? Where do they come from?

2. How specifically are restriction enzymes important to immunological work?

3. By what other names are restriction enzymes known? What role do they play in nature?

Section III
DISEASES AND DISORDERS

CHAPTER 16

BACTERIAL INFECTIONS IN SEXUALLY TRANSMITTED DISEASES

OUTLINE

- Venereal Syphilis: *Treponema pallidum*
  - Clinical Manifestation/Pathology
  - Immunology
  - Immunization Progress
- Laboratory Diagnosis
  - Non-Treponemal Tests
  - Standard Non-Treponemal Tests
  - Standard Treponemal Tests
  - Non-Standard Non-Treponemal and Treponemal Tests
- Gonorrhoea: *Neisseria gonorrhoeae*
  - Clinical Manifestation/Pathology
  - Immunology
  - Immunization
- Laboratory Diagnosis
  - Immunoassays to Detect Antigen
  - Ligase Chain Reaction Nucleic Acid Amplification Assay
- Genital Tract Infections: *Chlamydia trachomatis*
  - Energy Parasites
  - Clinical Manifestations/Pathology
  - Immunology
  - Immunization

- Laboratory Diagnosis
  - Optical Immunoassays for Antigen Detection
  - Mainstream Immunoassays for Antigen Detection
  - Nucleic Acid Amplification to Detect Antigen

OBJECTIVES

Upon completion of this chapter, the reader should be able to:

1. Provide a brief description of the bacteria that are causative agents of venereal syphilis, gonorrhea, and chlamydial genital tract infections.

2. Briefly describe the clinical manifestations of venereal syphilis, gonorrhea, and chlamydial genital tract infections.

3. Explain the role of the immune system and the effectors in host defense as a response to infections with bacteria that are the causative agents of venereal syphilis, gonorrhea, and chlamydial genital tract infections. As well, the reader should be able to describe the bacterial evasive strategies employed to establish infection.

4. Discuss the availability of vaccines, or the status of vaccine development, for the causative agents of venereal syphilis, gonorrhea, and chlamydial genital tract infections.

5. Describe laboratory tests that are available for diagnosis of each of these sexually transmitted bacteria. As well, the reader should be able to describe in detail one assay.

6. Compare and contrast molecular diagnostic tests based on nucleic acid amplification.

7. Compare and contrast molecular diagnostic tests based on signal amplification.

8. Compare and contrast the southern blot, northern blot, and western blot techniques.

9. Describe the role of PCR, southern blotting, and western blotting in the clinical laboratory.

SUMMARY OF KEY POINTS

Venereal syphilis or simply syphilis is a sexually transmitted disease caused by infection with *Treponema pallidum*, a spirochete bacterium that naturally infects humans and is transmitted from host to host. Intimate contact with an individual with a lesion is necessary for the transmission of this long, slender, spirally shaped bacterium. The organism enters the host through abraded skin or by penetrating mucous membranes.

Four clinical stages are recognized for untreated syphilis in adults: primary syphilis, secondary syphilis, latent syphilis, and tertiary syphilis each categorized by specific physiological manifestations reflecting the disease progression. Immune system evasion mechanisms for *T. pallidum* are poorly understood. Studies on these processes focus on phagocytosis and complement activation. Since *T. pallidum* becomes established in many hosts it must have evolved mechanisms to foil the immune system, and antibodies to specific *T. pallidum* proteins are produced in the immune response. The outer membrane protein and the endoflagellar protein can be detected suggesting these proteins have protective epitopes, so these proteins have been the focus for vaccine development.

Serological tests for syphilis diagnosis are based on antigen/antibody interactions, and there are two antibodies produced during infection with *T. pallidum*: antilipoidal antibodies (anti-cardiolipin antibodies or non-treponemal antibodies) and anti-*T. pallidum* antibodies (treponemal antibodies). The tests for diagnosis of syphilis are referred to as non-treponemal or treponemal tests in recognition of the type of antibodies detected in each test. Non-treponemal tests are screening procedures for syphilis, and these antibodies detected are called reagin antibodies. The Center for Disease Control (CDC) approves the rapid plasma reagin test (RPR), the untreated serum reagin test (USR), the toluidine red unheated serum test (TRUST), and the venereal disease research laboratory test (VDRL); flocculation is the end point for all these tests.

Treponemal tests are confirmatory tests for the diagnosis of syphilis such as the *Treponema pallidum* hemagglutination assay (TPHA), also known as microhemagglutination assay for *T. pallidum* (MHA-TP) or hemagglutination treponemal test for syphilis (HATTS). The two most commonly used assays in the clinical laboratory are the fluorescent treponemal antibody absorbed (FTA-ABS) test and the *T. pallidum* hemagglutination assay (TPHA). A number of non-standard treponemal and non-treponemal assays have been worked on, and one of the most promising assays is ELISA.

Gonorrhea is a disease usually transmitted by direct sexual contact and the genital tract is predominantly affected following contact with an infected individual; the causative agent is *Neisseria gonorrhoeae*. In most people, the disease is limiting and resolves quickly within about a month; without pharmacological intervention around one percent of infected males develop serious complications of the urethra, and 10–15% of untreated women develop pelvic inflammatory disease (PID). *N. gonorrhoeae*'s virulence is associated with surface proteins allowing the organism to attach to mucosal cell surfaces and enter the submucosa. The destruction of the organism via immunological mechanisms involves B cells making antibodies and complement activation. An effective vaccine for *N. gonorrhoeae* remains a challenge, although a number of approaches are currently under investigation.

Immunoassays or ligase chain reaction nucleic acid amplification technique (LCR) is used in diagnosis of *N. gonorrhoeae*. Two distinct phases of LCR are seen: probes target *N. gonorrhoeae* DNA for amplification in an automated thermal recycler, and the amplified product is detected using an automated enzyme immunoassay.

The most commonly transmitted disease in North America causing genital tract infections in humans is *Chlamydia trachomatis*. For many, the initial infection is asymptomatic, but severe disease can lead to infertility. *C. trachomatis* gains entry into susceptible host columnar epithelial cells by attaching to cell surface molecules with adhesive properties; one of the major adhesive molecules is the major outer membrane protein (MOMP), which serves as a target for antibody production and now for vaccine research. *C. trachomatis* is taken into endocytic vacuoles where it is changed from the elementary body form into the reticulate form and multiplies. The reticulate form remains in the endocytic vacuole to proliferate and ultimately to differentiate back to the elementary form and be released into the extracellular environment.

Long-term immunity to *C. trachomatis* does not accompany the strong humoral and cellular immune responses produced. The organism seems to persist in the host in a non-replicating form, and survives the effects of normally destructive lysosomal enzymes due to evolution of a mechanism preventing the fusion of lysosomes to the phagosome. The phagolysosome therefore does not form and so the organism thrives inside the endocytic vacuole. A vaccine would be beneficial, given the complications like blindness or infertility, but these studies are still in progress.

Culture or direct examination are not suitable for population screening, which is appropriate for this most commonly transmitted sexual disease in North America; and serological approaches have not proven effective for diagnosis of acute infections while they are of value for chronic infections and sero-epidemiological studies. Urine samples instead of invasive methods for specimens in the amplification assays may encourage asymptomatic high risk individuals to be tested for *C. trachomatis*. Amplification assays using either the nucleic acid or the signal are more sensitive and specific than those described in the antigen detection approach. Transcription-Mediated Amplification assay is performed using urine samples, endocervical (female) or urethral (male) swabs. Basic approach in this test is the amplification of a sequence of the *C. trachomatis* ribosomal RNA (rRNA). The amplified products (amplicons) are detected using an acridinium ester labeled DNA oligonucleotide probe in what is called the hybridization protection detection system.

REVIEW OF KEY TERMS AND ABBREVIATIONS

Matching: Match the key term in the left column with the definition in the right column.

1. _____ anti-lipoidal antibodies

2. _____ anti-*T. pallidum* antibodies

3. _____ cardiolipin

4. _____ chancre

5. _____ *Chlamydia trachomatis*

6. _____ columnar epithelial cells

7. _____ congenital syphilis

8. _____ DNA vaccine

9. _____ elementary bodies

10. _____ endocytic vacuoles

11. _____ endoflagellar protein

12. _____ factor H

13. _____ gonorrhea

14. _____ iron-binding proteins

15. _____ lipoprotein H8

16. _____ mucosal immunity

17. _____ Por

18. _____ reticulate bodies

19. _____ sialic acid

20. _____ trachoma

21. _____ ___ OMP

a) gram negative intracellular bacterium

b) in outer membrane unique to *Neisseria sp.*

c) *T. pallidum* from infected mother to fetus

d) *Neisseria*; usually from direct sexual contact

e) vaccines for *Chlamydia* must induce this

f) non-treponemal antibodies (anti-cardiolipin)

g) TpN19; outer membrane protein

h) extracellular, infectious form of *C. trachomatis*

i) modified sugar residue present in membrane

j) prevent growth and virulence of *Neisseria*

k) present in normal and treponemes; hapten

l) one of purified OMP proteins put into liposome

m) sialic acid binds it, blocks alternative pathway

n) leading cause of blindness in third world

o) potentially activate cellular and humoral immune response

p) TpN36; one protein candidate for vaccine

q) elementary bodies internalized here to convert

r) ulcerated lesion from *T. pallidum* entry

s) treponemal antibodies

t) undergo division; energy parasites of *Chlamydia*

u) *C. trachomatis* gains host entry here

Definitions: Write the definition of each of the following words or terms.

1. CCR5 _____

   _____

2. granulomatous _____

   _____

3. cardiolipin _____

   _____

4. delayed type hypersensitivity _____

   _____

5. seroconverted _____

   _____

6. reagin antibodies _____

   _____

7. TPI _____

   _____

8. western blotting _____

   _____

9. asymptomatic _____

   _____

10. neonates _____

   _____

11. opthalmia noenatorum _____

   _____

12. secretory IgA _____

   _____

13. energy parasites _____

   _____

REVIEW EXERCISES

True or False: Read each statement and decide if it is TRUE or FALSE. Place T or F on the line before each statement.

1. _____   Syphilis is caused by a spirochete.

2. _____   The latent syphilis stage is characterized by granulomatous lesions of the skin, bone, or viscera.

3. _____   Gonorrhea is caused by an intracellular bacterium infecting mucosal tissues.

4. _____   The predominant antibody formed in mucosal immunity is IgA.

Fill in the Blank: Complete the following sentences on the immune system by filling in the missing word or words.

1. _____ is a sexually transmitted disease caused by infection with a spirochete.

2. Infected mothers can spread syphilis to their unborn fetuses, which leads to _____ syphilis.

3. The lesion at the site of entry in primary syphilis is called a _____ .

4. Non-treponemal antibodies are also called _____ antibodies.

5. Sialic acid (modified sugar residue present in membrane) is known to bind _____ .

Multiple Choice: Choose the best answer.

1. Functions as T cell growth factor.

   a. interferon gamma
   b. interleukin-1
   c. interleukin-2
   d. type 2 cytokines
   e. C3b

2. A treponemal protein targeted for candidate vaccines.

   a. outer membrane protein
   b. protein A
   c. ubiquitin
   d. MHC
   e. seroconverted antibodies

3. Non-treponemal tests are syphilis diagnostic procedures that

   a. monitor efficacy of therapy.
   b. screen.
   c. confirm.
   d. b and c.
   e. a and b.

4. Gram negative bacteria causative agent of gonorrhea.

   a. *Treponema*
   b. *Neisseria*
   c. *Candida*
   d. *Chlamydia*
   e. *T. pallidum*

CASE STUDY

You come across a case in the hospital library for a class report. The subject experiences a burning sensation upon urination, and a yellowish green pus-like discharge from the urethra.

1. What sexually transmitted disease does the subject probably have? (What is the subject's sex? How can you tell?)

2. Describe the organism responsible for this infection, and detail how it attacks humans. What is the effect on the immune system, and why?

3. Is there a vaccine for this? Why or why not? What immunoassays are available to detect or diagnose this disease? How do they work?

CHAPTER 17

UPPER RESPIRATORY TRACT BACTERIAL INFECTIONS

OUTLINE

- Atypical Pneumonia: *Mycoplasma pneumoniae*
  - Clinical Manifestations/Pathology
  - Immunology
  - Immunization Progress
  - Laboratory Diagnosis
- Streptococcal Infections: *Streptococcaceae*
  - Lancefield Classification
  - Clinical Manifestations
  - Pathogenic Factors
  - Immunology
  - Immunization Progress
  - Laboratory Diagnosis
- Whooping Cough: *Bordetella pertussis*
  - Clinical Manifestations/Pathology
  - Immunology
  - Immunization
  - Laboratory Diagnosis

OBJECTIVES

Upon completion of this chapter, the reader should be able to:

1. Provide a brief description of the bacteria that are causative agents of atypical pneumonia, streptococcal infections, and whooping cough.

2. Briefly describe the clinical manifestations of atypical pneumonia, streptococcal infections, and whooping cough.

3. Explain the role of the immune system and the effectors in host defense as a response to infections with bacteria that are causative agents of atypical pneumonia, streptococcal infections, and whooping cough. As well, the reader should be able to describe the bacterial evasive strategies employed to establish infection.

4. Discuss the availability of vaccines, or the status of vaccine development, for the causative agents of atypical pneumonia, streptococcal infections, and whooping cough.

5. Describe laboratory tests that are available for diagnosis of each of these bacteria.

SUMMARY OF KEY POINTS

The causative agent of primary atypical pneumonia and tracheobronchitis is *Mycoplasma pneumoniae*, an extracellular bacterium with a single triple-layered membrane, which is very contagious and spread from person to person via respiratory secretions through households and other groups living in close contact. This disease is often called "walking pneumonia" because many infected individuals continue to work or go to school despite the malaise associated with *M. pneumoniae*, and about 60% of people infected with it develop cold agglutinins, which are IgM antibodies reactive to glycophorin (Ii antigen) present on human erythrocytes.

While *M. pneumoniae* can be cultured or isolated from sputum or nasopharyngeal swabs, these organisms are fastidious and therefore hard to culture, with a positive diagnosis requiring weeks of culture. The polymerase chain reaction (PCR) has potential for rapid diagnosis, although amplification techniques like PCR are not standard. Four types of serological tests, which have become standard for diagnosis, are now available commercially: the enzyme linked immunosorbent assay (ELISA), indirect fluorescent antibody test (IFA), complement fixation (CF), and cold agglutinin antibody titer tests.

Pathogenic streptococci bacteria cause streptococcal infections, although there are streptococci that are not pathogenic; and, to distinguish the species within the genus schemes have been devised such as the ability to lyse (or not lyse) red blood cells when grown on agar, and the Lancefield classification based on the antigenic characteristics of carbohydrate antigens found within walls of the streptococci.

Streptolysins, produced by some streptococci, cause hemolysis, and their actions categorize streptococci as beta-hemolytic (clear zone produced on agar plate or lysis of red blood cells), alpha-hemolytic (culture with greenish coloration due to partial hydrolysis), or non-hemolytic (red blood cells are not lysed).

Twenty-one different groups of C carbohydrate antigen are found within streptococcal walls (Lancefield classification), but only Groups A, B, C, D, F, and G contain human pathogens. Some common human pathogens include *S. pyogenes* (Group A, beta-hemolytic), *S. agalactiae* (Group B, beta-hemolytic), and *S. pneumoniae* (alpha-hemolytic) which does not express the C carbohydrate.

S. pyogenes causes a wide range of diseases and conditions including pharyngitis (strep throat), associated complications of pharyngitis such as rheumatic fever, necrotizing fasciitis, and toxic shock syndrome. Its pathogenicity is because the organism synthesizes virulence factors including lipoteichoic acid, M proteins, streptokinase, C5a peptidase, hyaluronidase, immunoglobulin-binding proteins, and some Group A strain toxins referred to as streptococcal pyrogenic exotoxins (SPEs A, B, C, and F). Flesh-eating bacteria represent some strains of *S. pyogenes*, which make SPE toxins causing necrotizing fasciitis (NF) progressively destroying host fascia and fat; and, streptococcal toxic shock syndrome is also associated with SPEs functioning as superantigens.

Adaptive immune responses to microbes, including streptococci, involve macrophages, dendritic cells, B cells, and T cells. Any organism not successfully removed at point of entry may spread through lymph capillaries, lymph, and the circulatory system. Development of effective vaccines focuses on investigating mechanisms by which bacteria invade hosts, virulence factors establishing the infection, and host factors altering the course of infection. Recombinant technology progress and the successful generation of protective immunity in response to selective epitopes of the M proteins have promoted phase I clinical trials for Group A streptococci.

Genetic probe techniques allow detection of *S. pyogenes* sequences in rRNA, rather than antigens of streptococci. Serological tests are predicated on detection of antibodies to streptolysin O (ASO), but antibodies to DNAses are also used for diagnosis, especially for post-streptococcal acute glomerulonephritis after skin infections. Direct recognition and/or culture of streptococcal antigens make up many laboratory tests for *S. pyogenes* infection.

Pertussis or whooping cough is caused by *Bordetella pertussis*, which is transmitted by aerosol droplets and is very contagious. *B. pertussis* has a tropism for ciliated epithelial cells of the respiratory tract whereby the cilia are immobilized. Virulence factors of *B. pertussis* include cell surface adhesins and secreted toxins. Toxins cause the most serious pathology, such as pertussis toxin, which is the most virulent and progressively destroys the ciliated epithelial cells.

B. pertussis infection has three stages: the first or catarrhal occurs one to three weeks after infection and includes red eyes, runny nose, mild cough, sneezing, and fever; the second or paroxysmal is characterized by violent coughing accompanied by a whooping sound; the third or convalescent extends up to six months. The immune system onslaught following infection with pertussis includes phagocytes, B cells, and CD4+ T cells, but *B. pertussis* has evolved strategies to survive, such as by production of adhesive molecules that bind and inactivate cilia and the prevention of lysosomal fusion with phagosomes. Classic pertussis vaccine is a cellular vaccine, made up of killed or partially detoxified whole *B. pertussis* organisms, which while being effective is also associated with adverse side effects. Most recent vaccines do not use whole organisms, but rather use a complex of purified or recombinant *B. pertussis* proteins, and these vaccines are called acellular.

Direct fluorescent antibody staining in clinical specimens can accomplish diagnosis of *B. pertussis*, and amplification techniques are replacing culture and DFA. Polymerase chain reaction (PCR) followed by nucleic acid hybridization for detection of amplicons are both more sensitive than DFA, but the efficacy of PCR depends on the primers selected for the amplification.

Rapid serological tests for widespread screening in developing countries would be beneficial, so investigations of enzyme linked immunoassays (ELISA) to detect the presence of anti-pertussis toxin IgG or IgA antibodies are being evaluated. Comparison of acute and convalescent sera is requisite for these tests. Passive hemagglutination is also being analyzed as a potential for widespread screening.

REVIEW OF KEY TERMS AND ABBREVIATIONS

Matching: Match the key term in the left column with the definition in the right column.

1. _____ acellular vaccine

2. _____ adhesive protein

3. _____ atypical pneumonia

4. _____ C carbohydrate

5. _____ carboxy terminus

6. _____ cellular vaccine

7. _____ cold agglutinins

8. _____ complement fixation

9. _____ contagious

10. _____ DNAse

11. _____ hyaluronidase

12. _____ hydrogen peroxide

13. _____ hypersensitivity

14. _____ M proteins

15. _____ necrotizing fasciitis

16. _____ nonhemolytic

17. _____ pharyngitis

18. _____ streptokinase

19. _____ tropism

20. _____ virulence factor

21. _____ digoxigenin

a) IgM antibodies reactive with glycophorin in erythrocytes

b) disease: host's fascia and fat are progressively destroyed

c) acute reaction to a particular substance

d) an enzyme that degrades DNA

e) dimeric surface proteins; form fringelike appearance

f) secretion initiating inflammatory response

g) attraction to a particular thing

h) *Streptococci* that do not lyse red blood cells

i) consists of killed or partially detoxified organisms

j) label on nucleotides used in PCR test for *M. pneumoniae*

k) an enzyme that dissolves blood clots

l) contributes to intensity of disease

m) consists of purified or recombinant proteins

n) strep throat

o) method for serological testing for *M. pneumoniae*

p) present in cell wall of nearly all *Streptococci*

q) presents like a viral infection; walking pneumonia

r) breaks down hyaluronic acid; spreading factor

s) one end of a protein

t) specialized filamentous tip characteristic of *M. pneumoniae*

u) easily spread from person to person

Definitions: Write the definition of each of the following words or terms.

1. acellular vaccine _____

_____

2. atypical pneumonia _____

_____

3. *Bordetella pertussis* _____

_____

4. catarrhal _____

_____

5. cilia _____

_____

6. cold agglutinins _____

_____

7. complement fixation _____

_____

8. convalescent _____

_____

9. GASD _____

_____

10. filamentous hemagglutinin _____

_____

11. Lancefield _____

_____

12. *Mycoplasma pneumoniae* _____

_____

13. walking pneumonia _____

_____

REVIEW EXERCISES

True or False: Read each statement and decide if it is TRUE or FALSE. Place T or F on the line before each statement.

1. _____ Reinfection of *Mycoplasma* is not common, and they are extracellular.

2. _____ Attachment is required for productive infection with *M. pneumoniae*.

3. _____ Streptolysins are molecules responsible for red blood cell lysis.

4. _____ Arthritis is the most common infection of *Streptococcus pyogenes*.

5. _____ There are no cases of immunocompetent individuals getting NF.

Fill in the Blank: Complete the following sentences on the immune system by filling in the missing word or words.

1. _____ is the causative agent of primary atypical pneumonia.

2. *M. pneumoniae* is _____ and spreads via respiratory secretions.

3. *M. pneumoniae* attaches to a glycoprotein on ciliated epithelial cells via a specialized filamentous tip containing an _____ .

4. The amplification test for detection of *M. pneumoniae* is the _____ .

5. One of the nucleotides in the PCR mixture is labeled with _____ .

Multiple Choice: Choose the best answer.

1. Classification scheme based on analysis of phenotypic characteristics of Streptococci.

   a. Lancefield
   b. virulence factors
   c. C carbohydrate
   d. DIG
   e. silicon assay surface technology

2. Causes most streptococcal infections in humans.

   a. *Mycoplasma pneumoniae*
   b. *Streptococcus agalactiae*
   c. *Streptococcus pyogenes*
   d. *Streptococcus pneumoniae*
   e. *Bordetella pertussis*

3. All are virulence factors of *S. pyogenes* except for

   a. M proteins.
   b. streptokinase.
   c. DNase.
   d. hyaluronidase.
   e. hyaluronic acid.

4. Sometimes referred to as spreading factor, because it facilitates the dissemination of *S. pyogenes* into tissues.

   a. C5a peptidase
   b. hyaluronidase
   c. hyaluronic acid
   d. M proteins
   e. SPEs

CRITICAL THINKING EXERCISE

Some nursing students are studying for a test on the cardiovascular system. Shock is one of their topics for study. They realize you may be able to help them understand some of the effects based on immune system responses that you just read in Chapter 17.

1. What kind of shock have you just read about in Chapter 17?

2. What pathogen and what toxins are responsible for most cases?

3. How might you link the signs and symptoms of this kind of shock to specific immune system responses?

CASE STUDY

Tom's wife, Amy, is a nursing assistant who has a very busy schedule, attending to a nine-year-old, going to the local community college, and working full-time to boot. For several weeks Amy has felt bad with a headache, chills, sore throat, and a non-productive dry cough. Amy thought it was just another viral "thing," and she managed to attend class and work full-time although at home she found herself not able to do much else. Tom finally convinced Amy that she was not getting any better, even though Amy pointed out her sputum was clear. Amy finally visited her family physician.

1. What did Amy most likely have? How can you tell?

2. What sort of complications can arise from this infection?

3. What sort of diagnostic means are available to detect the organism responsible for the infection or antibody tests?

CHAPTER 18

BACTERIAL INFECTIONS: TICK BORNE, ENTERIC, AND ZOONOTIC

OUTLINE

- Lyme Disease: *Borrelia burgdorferi*
  - Role of Ticks in Lyme Disease
  - Clinical Manifestations/Pathology
  - Immunology
  - Immunization
  - Laboratory Diagnosis
- Rocky Mountain Spotted Fever: *Rickettsia rickettsii*
  - Clinical Manifestations/Pathology
  - Immunology
  - Immunization Progress
  - Laboratory Diagnosis
- Leptospirosis: *Leptospira interrogans*
  - Clinical Manifestations/Pathology
  - Immunology
  - Immunization Progress
  - Laboratory Diagnosis
- Salmonellosis and Typhoid Fever: *Salmonella* species
  - Clinical Manifestations/Pathology
  - Immunology

- Immunization
- Laboratory Diagnosis

OBJECTIVES

Upon completion of this chapter, the reader should be able to:

1. Provide a brief description of the bacteria that are causative agents of Lyme disease, Rocky Mountain spotted fever, leptospirosis, and typhoid fever.

2. Briefly describe the clinical manifestations of Lyme disease, Rocky Mountain spotted fever, leptospirosis, and typhoid fever.

3. Explain the role of the immune system and the effectors in host defense as a response to infections with bacteria that are causative agents of Lyme disease, Rocky Mountain spotted fever, leptospirosis, and typhoid fever.

4. Describe the bacterial evasive strategies employed to establish infection.

5. Discuss the availability of vaccines, or the status of vaccine development, for the causative agents of Lyme disease, Rocky Mountain spotted fever, leptospirosis, and typhoid fever.

6. Describe laboratory tests that are available for diagnosis of each of these bacteria. As well, the reader should be able to describe, in detail, at least one diagnostic assay.

SUMMARY OF KEY POINTS

The causative agent of Lyme disease, so named to reflect the town of Lyme, Connecticut, where the first cluster of cases was documented is *Borrelia burgdorferi*. Humans pick up this bacterium from hard ticks, or arthropods in the same class as mites, that belong to the *Ixodes* genus. Hard ticks have four life stages: egg, larvae, nymph, and adult. The nymph stage is the source of most infections because the nymphs are very small and are able to attach to a host for prolonged periods without detection. Untreated *B. burgdorferi* infections may persist months or years even with a vigorous immune response due to antigenic variation. Antigenic variation (sequences within genes are changed during infection) is one of the mechanisms by which *B. burgdorferi* may evade destruction. The protein genetically altered after infection is a cell surface lipoprotein, VLsE (Variable major protein-Like Sequence, Expressed), which after an immune response is generated to one version of the VLsE, a different version is produced.

LYMErix vaccine is a transmission-blocking vaccine in which antibodies produced block transmission of the bacterium to the human when the infected tick takes up the antibodies during a blood meal. The antibodies bind to *B. burgdorferi* in the tick's midgut and prevent migration to the salivary glands, and because the transmission is typically by tick saliva this prevents transmission of the bacteria when the tick feeds on a host.

Serological testing, despite not being optimally sensitive or specific, is the main laboratory focus with Lyme disease. The Centers for Disease Control and Prevention (CDC) recommends a two-tier testing system in which positive or uncertain serological tests be followed by a western blot. Serological tests for *B. burgdorferi* antibodies include the indirect fluorescent antibody assays (IFA), enzyme immunoassay (EIA), complement fixation (CF), and the western blot.

Rickettsia rickettsii, an intracellular bacterium, causes Rocky Mountain spotted fever (RMSF). When an infected tick (the dog tick is the principal eastern region vector) attaches to the skin for several hours, humans become hosts for *R. rickettsii*. Cellular immunity and Type 1 cytokines (interferon gamma) play a larger role in host immunity than humoral immunity because T cells secrete interferon gamma, which binds to phagocyte receptors stimulating nitric oxide production in the cytosol. Nitric oxide is cytotoxic to *R. rickettsii*. Vaccine research has centered on outer membrane proteins mediating adhesion of *R. rickettsii* to host cells, and antibodies to the outer membrane protein A have been shown to block attachment *in vitro*. A subunit vaccine containing outer major surface proteins has thus been promoted for animal studies.

RMSF is diagnosed usually without laboratory analysis, based instead on clinical presentations and a history of a patient's exposure to ticks or travel to locations where infections have occurred. Therapy should be started long before laboratory tests are available, so immediate diagnosis is important. Serological tests use purified or recombinant *R. rickettsii* proteins as antigens: indirect immunofluorescent antibody, enzyme immunoassay latex agglutination, and complement fixation. The Weil-Felix test formed the basis for diagnosis of rickettsial infections for more than fifty years, and the latex agglutination test, Latex-*R-rickettsii*, is a commercially available test intended to replace the Weil-Felix test.

Leptospira interrogans, an aerobic spirochete with worldwide distribution, is a zoonosis causing leptospirosis. (A zoonosis refers to an infectious disease in humans caused by an organism whose natural reservoir is a non-human animal.) Leptospirosis has two stages: a septicemic stage and an immunologic stage. The septicemia stage presents as fever, myalgia, and headache, and the immunological stage manifests as either anicteric leptospirosis (self-limiting disease but may persist for weeks or months) or icteric leptospirosis (ten percent develop this more severe form of the disease, also called Weil's disease).

Direct contact with urine from infected animals transmits *L. interrogans* to humans, or contact with water contaminated with animal urine containing the leptospires can also be a source of infection. Opsonin-mediated phagocytosis and complement-mediated lysis are primary host defense mechanisms. Opsonins are complement fragments C3b and IgG antibodies. No vaccine exists in North America at present for *L. interrogans*, although some parts of Europe and Asia have a vaccine available for individuals at high risk for infection.

Diagnosis is made on serological studies or demonstration of the organism in samples of clinical fluids. Current assays are LEPTO Lateral Flow and LEPTO Dri-Dot, both of which are commercially available.

Salmonellosis refers to collective clinical manifestations caused by intestinal bacterial pathogens, most disease in humans being produced by ten serotypes, and of these *Salmonella typhi* and *S. enteritidis* are major causes of human disease. *S. typhi* produces the SpiC protein, which prevents fusion of the lysosome with the phagosome, thus making *S. typhi* a successful pathogen resisting destruction. Whole, inactivated cell vaccines are licensed for intradermal injection against *S. typhi*, but are not often used because of adverse reactions in many of those vaccinated, and protection is not complete. Oral administration of killed whole cell preparations is an alternative mode of vaccine delivery with none of the adverse effects associated with the intradermal injections, but only partial protection is thus afforded.

Diagnosis of *S. typhi* is by detection in culture, and is the standard diagnosis method for typhoid fever. A chromogenic culture medium (CHROMager) essentially selective for *Salmonella sp.* has helped this process. Serological tests to measure antibodies have been available for years. The Widal agglutination test introduced over 100 years ago by F. Widal is commonly employed in developing countries. The counter-immunoelectrophoresis assay is also used. An enzyme immunoassay for IgM antibodies, using the DIP-S-TICK method is available from PanBioINDX, and the results of this test are available in minutes.

REVIEW OF KEY TERMS AND ABBREVIATIONS

Matching: Match the key term in the left column with the definition in the right column.

1. _____ antigenic variation

2. _____ attentuation

3. _____ cassettes

4. _____ DIP-S-TICK

5. _____ facial palsy

6. _____ gastroenteritis

7. _____ H antigen

8. _____ recovery phase

9. _____ K antigen

10. _____ Leptospirosis

11. _____ LYMErix

12. _____ nymph

13. _____ RMSF

14. _____ rOmpA

15. _____ salmonella

16. _____ septicemic stage

17. _____ SpiC protein

18. _____ spontaneous

19. _____ tick

20. _____ vascular collapse

21. _____ Vi antigen

a) paralysis of facial muscles

b) zoonosis caused by bacterium *Leptospira interrogans*

c) immunological phase

d) an outer membrane protein

e) gene sequences consistently changed during infection

f) immature adult form of the tick

g) vessels cannot adequately transport blood and nutrients

h) molecule used to serotype salmonella

i) infectious phase

j) disease caused by the bacteria *enterobacteriaceae*

k) mutations seeming to occur randomly, without stimulus

l) segments of the VLse

m) arthropod in same class as mites

n) disease caused by *Rickettsia rickettsii*

o) disorder of digestive and gastrointestinal tract

p) inhibits fusion of lysosomes with phagosome

q) enzyme immunoassay detects *S. typhi* IgM antibodies

r) purified antigen used as vaccination for typhoid

s) molecule used to serotype salmonella

t) vaccine used to prevent Lyme disease

u) weaken the virulence of a bacteria

Definitions: Write the definition of each of the following words or terms.

1. Anicteric leptospires _____

   _____

2. antigenic variation _____

   _____

3. *Borrelia burgdorferi* _____

   _____

4. bull's eye appearance _____

   _____

5. febrile agglutination test _____

   _____

6. FITC _____

   _____

7. icteric leptospires _____

   _____

8. LEPTO Dri-Dot test _____

   _____

9. LEPTO lateral flow test _____

   _____

10. Lyme disease _____

    _____

11. *Rickettsia rickettsii* _____

    _____

12. transmission blocking vaccine _____

    _____

13. Widal agglutination _____

    _____

REVIEW EXERCISES

True or False: Read each statement and decide if it is TRUE or FALSE. Place T or F on the line before each statement:

1. _____ Lyme disease is named after a town in Massachusetts.

2. _____ Tick saliva transmits bacteria or viruses during a blood meal.

3. _____ *B. burgdorferi* has a very sophisticated means of antigenic variation.

4. _____ *R. rickettsii* prevent infected cells from undergoing apoptosis.

5. _____ The natural reservoir is human in a zoonosis.

Fill in the Blank: Complete the following sentences on the immune system by filling in the missing word or words.

1. _____ is the causative agent of Lyme disease.

2. *Borrelia burgdorferi* is transmitted to humans via hard _____ in *Ixodes* genus.

3. Most common neurological symptom with Lyme disease is _____ .

4. _____ is a mechanism microbes use to escape destruction by the immune system.

5. Proteins associated with *B. burgdorferi* _____ are studied as candidate vaccines.

Multiple Choice: Choose the best answer.

1. All these are serological tests used for detection of antibodies to *B. burgdorferi* except

    a. indirect fluorescent antibody assays (IFA).
    b. complement fixation (CF).
    c. enzyme immunoassay (EIA).
    d. western blot.
    e. polymerase chain reaction (PCR).

2. Rocky mountain spotted fever is caused by an intracellular

    a. virus.
    b. bacterium.
    c. endosome.
    d. phagosome.
    e. fungus.

3. One of the outer membrane proteins shown to be critical for adhesion to host cells is

    a. rOmpA.
    b. filopodia.
    c. opsonin.
    d. OX-2 antigens.
    e. colloidal gold.

4. Plays more significant role in host immunity to *R. rickettsii*.

   a. humoral immunity
   b. cellular immunity
   c. phagolysosome
   d. apoptosis
   e. Proteus strains

CRITICAL THINKING EXERCISE

You overhear someone mentioning the term "accidental hosts" in the hall one day between classes. You have visions of a Gary Larson cartoon, but you consider the term seriously having just read Chapter 18. Later on a fellow student asks you about it.

1. What are *accidental* hosts as opposed to natural hosts? What is a zoonosis?

2. Which organism and disease in Chapter 18 is associated with humans as accidental hosts?

3. What other examples can you give of this phenomenon? How might this sort of transmission be of benefit to the infectious organism?

CASE STUDY

A well-known 65-year-old woman named Edith living all her life in a small urban center in the Midwest has been residing in a nursing home now for around three years. She has adjusted well, is healthy except for arthritis, and is an active part of the community there. This past weekend the nursing home had a celebration of its founding and there was a large dinner. On Tuesday following this weekend dinner Edith was extremely nauseous, had severe abdominal cramps and massive diarrhea. The staff physician immediately saw to Edith's condition as well as to a majority of the individuals in the nursing home.

1. Edith is presenting signs and symptoms of what sort of infection? What treatment will the physician most probably decide upon for Edith and why?

2. What organism and species is most certainly the culprit in Edith's situation?

3. What is the most serious complication of this infection? How long might it take for complete resolution? What is responsible for the pathology observed? What evasive mechanisms exist for this organism to protect it from the immune system?

CHAPTER 19

HEPATITIS

OUTLINE

- The Causative Agents of Hepatitis
  - Hepatitis A Virus
  - Hepatitis B Virus
  - Hepatitis C Virus
- Clinical Manifestations/Pathology
  - Hepatitis A
  - Hepatitis B
  - Hepatitis C
- Immunology of Hepatitis Infections
  - Hepatitis A and Hepatitis B
  - Hepatitis C
- Immunization
  - Hepatitis A Vaccine
  - Hepatitis B Vaccine
  - Hepatitis C Vaccine Progress
- Laboratory Diagnosis
  - Hepatitis A
  - Hepatitis B
  - Hepatitis C

OBJECTIVES

Upon completion of this chapter, the reader should be able to:

1. Provide a brief description of the viruses that are causative agents of Hepatitis A, Hepatitis B, and Hepatitis C.

2. Briefly describe the clinical manifestations of Hepatitis A, Hepatitis B, and Hepatitis C.

3. Explain the role of the immune system and the effectors in host defense as a response to infections with viruses that are causative agents of Hepatitis A, Hepatitis B, and Hepatitis C.

4. Discuss the availability of vaccines, or the status of vaccine development, for the causative agents of Hepatitis A, Hepatitis B, and Hepatitis C.

5. Describe the laboratory tests that are available for diagnosis of Hepatitis A, Hepatitis B, and Hepatitis C.

SUMMARY OF KEY POINTS

Viral hepatitis is a systemic disease caused by Hepatitis A, Hepatitis B, and Hepatitis C viruses, although there are other viruses associated with acute hepatitis in which the liver is the main target. Viral hepatitis is a significant cause of morbidity and mortality worldwide.

Hepatitis A is transmitted via a fecal-oral route and person to person contact is the primary mode of transmission, so hepatitis A infections are common in countries where the sanitation is inadequate and water supplies are contaminated. Clinical symptoms of hepatitis A occur as early as two weeks, but as late as six weeks post infection, and the clinical symptoms usually resolve within one to two months of onset. Natural killer cells or CD8+ T cells destroy virally-infected cells, while B cell activation and production of IgM and IgG antibodies also occurs. The antibodies can bind to the virus before it enters cells and prevent the virus from infecting hepatocytes. The hepatitis A vaccine, Havrix, is an inactivated hepatitis A virus given in two doses that induces high titers of antibodies in around 99% of vaccine recipients after the second dose. There are techniques available to measure HAV infection, some measuring the presence of HAV antigen; others measure the anti-hepatitis antibody in serum. Serological diagnostic tests are based on IgG (previous infection) or IgM (recent infection) antibody detection.

Hepatitis B antigens of clinical significance are the antigenically complex surface antigen, HBsAg, and HBeAg, a truncated form of HBcAg. HBeAg is proteolytically cleaved from HBcAg, but the two peptides have different antigen specificities. Laboratory tests detecting anti-HBc, anti-HBs, or anti-HBe antibodies are used to tell the stage of infection. In clinical diagnosis of an active infection with HBV, the patient's serum would have a high serum level of HBsAg, and anti-HBc antibodies.

HBV is found in all bodily fluids including blood, saliva, semen, and breast milk, and transmission is through direct contact with these fluids. Incubation for HBV is six weeks to six months. Once again, natural killer cells and CD8+ T cells destroy virally-infected cells, and infection with hepatitis B virus leads to production of IgM and IgG antibodies, which can bind to the virus before it can enter cells. There is a hepatitis B vaccine (Recombivax HB), that is a recombinant protein given in three doses. Diagnosis of hepatitis B infection is complex because the presence of various antibodies or viral proteins in the patient's serum/plasma sample varies depending on the time of diagnosis, relative to the time of infection.

Three particles, all of which are reactive with the anti-HBs antibody, are present in sera from individuals with hepatitis B: Dane particle (intact hepatitis virion), spherical non-infectious particles without the viral genome, and a tubular form that is also non-infectious. Commercial tests available for diagnosis of hepatitis B include fully automated tests, rapid one-step immunodiagnostic assays using latex agglutination, cassettes, membrane test strips, or dipsticks, and branched DNA (bDNA) technology and hybrid capture system.

Hepatitis C virus (HCV), the causative agent of non-A and non-B hepatitis, is classed into six principal genotypes referred to as clades, which respond differently to therapy. Primarily, most infections with HCV are transmitted by blood (sharing of needles, hemodialysis, and occupational exposure to blood). Infections with HCV are characterized by a long incubation (two to five months) and the majority infected do not develop overt clinical symptoms, although in symptomatic patients the clinical manifestations are similar but less severe than that of HBV.

It was not until 1996 that the putative hepatitis C virus was identified, so investigations with hepatitis C are recent and demonstrate virus specific antibodies present in infected individuals. Hepatitis C specific CD8+ T cells have been isolated from the liver, and to date there is no vaccine against hepatitis C. Two types of tests are available for HCV: serological tests based on enzyme immunoassay technology and confirmatory western blot (immunoblotting), and molecular technology used to assess the level of HCV particles or to identify the HCV clade.

REVIEW OF KEY TERMS AND ABBREVIATIONS

Matching: Match the key term in the left column with the definition in the right column.

1. _____ anti-HBs antibody

2. _____ clades

3. _____ Dane particle

4. _____ E1

5. _____ E2

6. _____ gamma globulins

7. _____ HbcAg

8. _____ HbeAg

9. _____ HbsAg

10. _____ viral hepatitis

a) intact infectious hepatitis B virion

b) core protein antigen in HBV infection

c) HCV membrane binding to cell surface molecule CD81

d) truncated form of HbcAg in HBV infection

e) principle genotypes of HCV

f) complex surface antigen in HBV infection

g) non-infectious particles not containing HBV genome

h) systemic disease in which the liver is the main target

i) protein antibodies found in human plasma cells

j) HCV membrane protein

Definitions: Write the definition of each of the following words or terms.

1. Anti-HBs antibody _____

_____

2. clades _____

_____

3. Dane particle _____

_____

4. E1 _____

_____

5. E2 _____

_____

6. gamma globulins _____

_____

7. HAV _____

_____

8. HBV _____

_____

9. HCV _____

_____

REVIEW EXERCISES

True or False: Read each statement and decide if it is TRUE or FALSE. Place T or F on the line before each statement.

1. _____ Hepatitis A virus, single stranded RNA, is a member of *Picornaviridae*.

2. _____ Hepatitis B virus, enveloped DNA, is a member of *Hepadnaviridae*.

3. _____ Hepatitis C, enveloped single strand RNA, is a member of *Flaviviridae*.

4. _____ Virally infected cells are killed by natural killer cells.

5. _____ Persistence of hepatitis C virus is related to its quick mutation rate.

Fill in the Blank: Complete the following sentences on the immune system by filling in the missing word or words.

1. There are six principal genotypes of HCV referred to as _____ .

2. The _____ route is the primary transmission for hepatitis A.

3. Passive immunization with pooled human _____ was possible before the development of a vaccine for hepatitis A for travelers to high-risk areas.

4. The _____ is the intact infectious hepatitis B virion.

5. _____ transmission is by direct contact with bodily fluids such as blood.

Multiple Choice: Choose the best answer.

1. Approach to use transgenic plants as vectors for hepatitis candidate vaccines.

   a. opsonin-mediated
   b. ELISA
   c. edible vaccines
   d. natural killer cells
   e. blood transfusion

2. Potential sources of HCV are

   a. nursing (breast milk).
   b. hemodialysis.
   c. cattle.
   d. domestic cat.
   e. blood transfusion after 1990.

3. Fecal/oral route is the primary transmission of infection by this causative agent of hepatitis.

   a. HCV and HBV
   b. HBV only
   c. HCV and HAV
   d. HCV only
   e. HAV only

4. This cell type destroys virally infected cells (*hint*: part of adaptive immune response).

   a. natural killer cells
   b. CD8+ T cells
   c. CD4+ T cells
   d. B cells
   e. eosinophils

CRITICAL THINKING/CASE STUDY EXERCISE

While taking a contemporary justice course at school you meet an individual who freely admits to the class that he has been arrested on drug charges in the past. This person has a skin rash, which is hard not to notice. He also makes a comment after an anatomy class on the urinary system about how dark his urine is. You note that he has skin and eyes with a light yellow tinge, and you recall liver function and what bilirubin is from anatomy, too. Other symptoms are fatigue, nausea, anorexia (loss of appetite), and joint pain, and he casually says he feels like he has the "flu" or something.

1. What presumptive diagnosis would you make based upon your reading of Chapter 19? How might this infection have been transmitted?

2. What is the main site of infection for this individual? What is the incubation time?

3. How does tissue damage occur in this infectious disease?

CHAPTER 20

MEASLES, MUMPS, RUBELLA, AND VARICELLA

OUTLINE

- Measles
  - Clinical Manifestations/Pathology
  - Immunology
  - Immunization
  - Laboratory Diagnosis
- Mumps
  - Clinical Manifestations/Pathology
  - Immunology
  - Immunization
  - Laboratory Diagnosis
- Rubella
  - Clinical Manifestations/Pathology
  - Immunology
  - Immunization
  - Laboratory Diagnosis
- Varicella
  - Clinical Manifestations/Pathology
  - Immunology
  - Immunization
  - Laboratory Diagnosis

OBJECTIVES

Upon completion of this chapter, the reader should be able to:

1. Provide a brief description of the viruses that are causative agents of measles. mumps, rubella, and varicella.

2. Briefly describe the clinical manifestations of measles, mumps, rubella, and varicella.

3. Explain the role of the immune system and the effectors in host defense as a response to infections with viruses that are causative agents of measles, mumps, rubella, and varicella.

4. Discuss the availability of vaccines, or the status of vaccine development, for the causative agents of measles, mumps, rubella, and varicella.

5. Describe laboratory tests that are available for diagnosis of each of measles, mumps, rubella, and varicella.

SUMMARY OF KEY POINTS

Measles is highly contagious, caused by the measles virus, and presents with runny nose, fever, cough, sneezing, and photophobia as an early symptom. It is referred to as red measles (rubeola) to distinguish it from German measles (rubella). Koplik's spots or spots on the mouth epithelium are diagnostic for measles, although some patients do not develop these spots. There are humoral and cellular immune responses to measles, and both the absolute numbers of CD4+ and CD8+ T cells is decreased while the ratio of the two subsets remains constant. There are monovalent (Attenuvax) and trivalent forms for the measles vaccine, which is made up of attenuated measles virus, typically administered as a trivalent vaccine in the MMR (measles, mumps, and rubella) vaccine. Clinical symptoms can be used for presumptive diagnosis, but the presence of IgM is diagnostic for a recent infection and confirmation requires either a positive serological test or isolation of the virus from samples. For detection of anti-measles IgM, IgG, or IgA antibodies, various enzyme linked immunosorbent assays (ELISA) are available. Indirect antibody tests are also used for detection of anti-measles antibodies in serum.

Mumps virus is the causative agent of the infectious disease, mumps, and the virus is usually transmitted by droplets via the upper respiratory route in which primary viral replication occurs in the mucosal epithelium and lymphocytes in that region. Dissemination of the virus to the salivary glands (parotids) and the central nervous system follows viral replication, and both humoral (extracellular virus) and cellular (intracellular virus) immune components participate in response to the viral infection. The immune system eliminates the viral infection, once the virus is sequestered within the cell, by destroying the cell. Natural killer cells and CD8+ T cells are the two types of cytotoxic cells. Attenuated mumps virus vaccine (Mumpsvax) is available as both monovalent and a trivalent vaccine, but it is usually administered as the trivalent form with the measles (Attenuvax) and rubella (Meruvax II) vaccines. Diagnosis of mumps is made with emphasis on the swelling of the parotid glands. Clinical specimens may be blood, urine, saliva, or cerebral spinal fluid. Urine samples may contain viral particles for two weeks post onset of symptoms, and the indirect immunofluorescent antibody test as well as the enzyme immunoassays (ELISA and ELFA) are useful in confirmation of a diagnosis of mumps.

Rubella, also known as German measles and not to be confused with rubeola or red measles, is transmitted by direct contact with nasopharyngeal secretions of infected individuals. Rubella is usually a mild disease characterized by a discrete pink maculopapular rash appearing on the face that spreads to the trunk and extremities. Rubella is serious if acquired during the first trimester of pregnancy because the virus may spread to the fetus through the placenta and result in congenital rubella syndrome.

This congenital rubella syndrome can affect fetal development and lead to birth defects such as cardiac anomalies, deafness, and mental retardation. Cellular and humoral immunity both play a role in the immune response to rubella virus. The most widely used vaccine is a component of the trivalent MMR (measles, mumps, and rubella) vaccine, but the monovalent vaccine is an attenuated rubella virus sold under the name of Meruvax II. Confirmation of a rubella diagnosis may be made by enzyme immunoassays using different platforms. EIAs, passive agglutination, and immunofluorescence are also used. Antibodies to the E1, E2, or nucleocapsid protein C are the basis of these serological tests. Agglutination is a quick and inexpensive screening method for rubella antibodies, and amplification techniques are useful for congenital rubella syndrome diagnosis.

Varicella or chicken-pox is a clinical manifestation of infection with the varicella-zoster virus, which may persist in a latent form in nerves (dorsal root ganglion or extra medullary cranial ganglia). Reactivation of latent varicella-zoster usually occurs in elderly or immunocompromised individuals, and leads to zoster (shingles). Varicella-zoster is highly contagious and the transmission is the result of direct contact with infected respiratory secretions released during sneezing and coughing; however, alternative contact with fluid from vesicular lesions, or fresh-contaminated discharge on clothing or other articles (fomites) may serve as vehicles for transmission.

Chicken-pox is usually benign in otherwise healthy (immunocompetent) children, with mainly cellular immune responses occurring that involve natural killer cells of innate immunity and cytotoxic CD8+ T cells of adaptive immunity. Both these mechanisms require the presence of cytokines derived from CD4+ T cells. B cell responses to viruses occur only when the virion is outside the cell. Varivax or an attenuated varicella virus has been available for use in healthy individuals since March 1995. Adults may need a second dose one to two months later for effective vaccination, and a tetravalent measles-mumps-rubella-varicella vaccine has recently been tested in children with similar seroconversion rates and reactions as those from the trivalent vaccine.

Commercially available ELISA tests are sensitive, simple, and useful for screening past infection or confirmation of clinical diagnosis if it is important to confirm the diagnosis or antibody titer before vaccination, although routine laboratory tests are not required. Acute phase blood samples are tested for IgG antibodies and compared with a convalescent phase sample collected about 14 days later to confirm diagnosis. Four-fold increases in antibody titer indicate recent infection.

Complications of varicella-zoster, although rare, are documented, such as encephalitis and varicella pneumonia. Viral presence or one of its products can be detected by immunofluorescence techniques, in situ hybridization, or the polymerase chain reaction (PCR). Since virus is not shed, its presence in tissue is diagnostic of infection.

REVIEW OF KEY TERMS AND ABBREVIATIONS

Matching: Match the key term in the left column with the definition in the right column.

1. _____ alkaline phosphatase

2. _____ Attenuvax

3. _____ chicken-pox

4. _____ fusion

5. _____ German measles

a) varicella-zoster virus infection; varicella

b) pipette-like device coated with inactivated mumps virus

c) vaccine for mumps

d) rare neurological complication of measles

e) protein associated with cell membrane in measles virus

6. _____ hemagglutinin

7. _____ Koplick's spots

8. _____ matrix

9. _____ measles

10. _____ Meruvax II

11. _____ mumps virus

12. _____ parotid glands

13. _____ varicella

14. _____ VZIG

15. _____ Varivax

16. _____ VIDAS

17. _____ rubella

18. _____ rubeola

19. _____ SPR

20. _____ SSPE

21. _____ Mumpsvax

f) vaccine for rubella

g) infection with varicella-zoster virus; chicken-pox

h) used to label anti-IgG antibodies in the ELFA test

i) vaccine for chicken-pox

j) enveloped virus in *paramyxoviridae* family

k) RNA virus of *togaviridae* family; German measles

l) vaccine for measles

m) protein associated with cell membrane in measles virus

n) commercial kit used to diagnose mumps

o) RNA virus of *togaviridae* family; rubella

p) very contagious, member of *paramyoxoviridae*; measles

q) highly contagious; *paramyoxoviridae*; rubeola

r) passive immunization for chicken-pox

s) small irregular red spots characteristic of measles

t) salivary glands; exocrine glands in the neck

u) protein associated with cell membrane in measles virus

Definitions: Write the definition of each of the following words or terms.

1. alkaline phosphatase _____

_____

2. Attenuvax _____

_____

3. chicken-pox _____

_____

4. congenital rubella syndrome _____

_____

5. fusion _____

_____

6. German measles _____

_____

7. hemagglutinin _____

_____

8. Koplick's spots _____

_____

9. measles _____

_____

10. mumps virus _____

_____

11. Reye's syndrome _____

_____

12. varicella _____

_____

13. subacute sclerosing panencephalitis _____

_____

REVIEW EXERCISES

True or False: Read each statement and decide if it is TRUE or FALSE. Place T or F on the line before each statement.

1. _____ Measles virus is an enveloped double stranded DNA virus.

2. _____ Mumps virus has a single stranded RNA genome encoding six mRNA.

3. _____ Natural killer cells are cytotoxic for virally infected autologous cells.

4. _____ Passive immunization comes from donors with high antibody titers.

5. _____ Reverse transcription of viral RNA makes complementary DNA.

Fill in the Blank: Complete the following sentences on the immune system by filling in the missing word or words.

1. A rare complication of measles is _____ .

2. _____ are cytotoxic for virally infected autologous cells.

3. Spots on the mouth epithelium are diagnostic for measles and are called _____ .

4. Passive immunization may reduce the severity of measles when _____ is given within 72 hours of exposure.

5. Mumps virus replication within infected cells is followed by dissemination of the virus to the _____ glands.

Multiple Choice: Choose the best answer.

1. Rare complication of varicella-zoster infections is

   a. encephalitis and pneumonia.
   b. subacute sclerosing panencephalitis.
   c. chicken-pox.
   d. shingles.
   e. influenza.

2. Cytotoxic component of innate immunity for virally infected autologous cells is

   a. CD4+ T cells.
   b. CD8+ T cells.
   c. natural killer cells.
   d. antibodies.
   e. plasma cells.

3. When administered it is referred to as passive immunization.

   a. immunoglobulin
   b. Attenuvax
   c. ELISA
   d. Mumpsvax
   e. transgenic plants as edible vaccines

4. Classic clinical diagnosis of mumps infection.

   a. isolation from saliva clinical specimens
   b. urine samples
   c. parotid glands swelling
   d. ELFA
   e. discrete pink maculopapular facial rash

CRITICAL THINKING EXERCISE

Your study group is reviewing Chapter 20. Sarah is talking about measles, but something she says lets Tom know that she probably is not distinguishing the types of measles. Tom is diplomatic and waits until complications of measles comes up as a topic, and then he interjects that there is a type of measles very dangerous for pregnant women.

1. Why does Tom mention the pregnancy danger? Which type of measles is Tom referring to and why?

2. What are the types of measles and how do you distinguish them? How would you make a diagnosis?

3. What sorts of tests are available to confirm a presumptive diagnosis? Are there vaccines available?

CASE STUDY

As a social worker you are helping some indigent families with young children get the health care that they so desperately need. Shockingly, many of the families have never even had their children vaccinated for one reason or other. You notice that one family has a 14-year-old son who is presenting the following signs and symptoms: fever, malaise, and myalgia. Furthermore, the boy seems to be wincing every time he swallows.

1. What is your presumptive diagnosis of the boy's illness? Why? What is the etiology (cause) and epidemiology (contagious spread and dissemination) of this condition?

2. What is the incubation period for this infection? Discuss the immunology of this infection, and the roles played by various immune system components.

3. What complications are possible, and which are maybe more critical in this specific situation with the 14-year-old boy? What immunization is available, and what laboratory tests will clinically diagnose this case?

CHAPTER 21

VIRUSES III

OUTLINE

- Adenovirus
  - Clinical Manifestations/Pathology
  - Immunology
  - Immunization
  - Laboratory Diagnosis
- Cytomegalovirus
  - Clinical Manifestations/Pathology
  - Immunology
  - Immunization Progress
  - Laboratory Diagnosis
- Epstein Barr Virus
  - Clinical Manifestations/Pathology
  - Immunology
  - Immunization Progress
  - Laboratory Diagnosis
- Influenza Virus
  - Function of HA and NA
  - Clinical Manifestations/Pathology
  - Immunology
  - Immunization
  - Laboratory Diagnosis

- Polio
  - Clinical Manifestations/Pathology
  - Immunology
  - Immunization
  - Laboratory Diagnosis

OBJECTIVES

Upon completion of this chapter, the reader should be able to:

1. Provide a brief description of the adenovirus, Epstein Barr virus, cytomegalovirus, influenza virus, and the poliovirus.

2. Briefly describe the clinical manifestations caused by infections with adenovirus, Epstein Barr virus, cytomegalovirus, influenza virus, and the poliovirus.

3. Explain the role of the immune system and the effectors in host defense as a response to infections with adenovirus, Epstein Barr virus, cytomegalovirus, influenza virus, and the poliovirus.

4. Discuss the availability of vaccines, or the status of vaccine development, for adenovirus, Epstein Barr virus, cytomegalovirus, influenza virus, and the poliovirus.

5. Describe the laboratory tests that are available for diagnosis of infection with adenovirus, Epstein Barr virus, cytomegalovirus, influenza virus, and the poliovirus.

SUMMARY OF KEY POINTS

Adenovirus, a common pathogen with most common serotypes causing infection in the upper respiratory tract, is transmitted via droplets when an infected person coughs or sneezes. Infections in immunocompromised individuals (T cell defects) can be very serious and even fatal, because the primary host defense mechanisms are the cytotoxic T cells. Oral delivery vaccines for mucosal immunity containing attenuated adenoviruses in a gelatin capsule are available to recruits, but an adenoviral vector is currently being tested for use in gene therapy trials and DNA vaccines. Antigen specific and serological tests are available.

Cytomegalovirus infections cause morbidity and mortality in immunocompromised patients, in which transmission of CMV requires contact with respiratory secretions or other body fluids including tears, feces, urine, and genital secretions, although CMV can be transmitted from mother to fetus or in transfusions of blood products without appropriate screening. CMV infections in the immunocompetent host are often asymptomatic, but CMV infection in the immunocompromised individual may result in extended fever, retinal infections (could lead to blindness), pneumonia, encephalitis, hepatitis, and gastrointestinal disease. Anti-CMV antibodies may reduce mortality rates for immunocompromised patients following bone marrow transplantation, as antibodies made during the immune response target CMV outside the cell. Cytotoxic CD8+ T cells and natural killer cells (both kill virally infected cells) are primary immunological effectors to get rid of CMV infections. However, CMV is able to hinder the expression of class I MHC/viral peptide complexes on the surface of infected cells thereby reducing the number of such complexes on the cell surface and reducing the efficacy of CD8+ T cells that target those complexes on infected cells. A CMV glycoprotein B subunit vaccine with an adjuvant, MF59, is a recent development, and laboratory diagnosis is based on detection of antibodies, CMV particles, or amplification tests.

Epstein Barr virus causes infectious mononucleosis and is a contributing factor in B cell malignancy, Burkitt's lymphoma, and nasopharyngeal carcinoma. EBV is infectious but not very contagious, initiated in the salivary glands, and it is present in saliva and disseminated in this way. This is the reason EBV is referred to as the *kissing disease*. EBV is found in circulating B cells and can be passed via blood. With no vaccine for EBV, a phase I clinical trial using Epstein Barr virus vaccine has been started.

EBV has evolved a way to prevent class I MHC/viral peptide complexes from being expressed on the infected cell's surface. EBV prevents hydrolysis of viral peptides to a size that fits into the class I MHC groove, so CD8+ T cells potential lytic ability is lowered since this is how they recognize the virally infected cell. Antibodies (from the B cell responses) are made to the viral capsid antigens, EBV early antigens, and EBV nuclear proteins, and they all play an important role in laboratory diagnosis. Heterophile antibodies are also made (tested for in the past by the classic Paul-Bunnell Davidsohn Differential Test), but more rapid tests to detect heterophile antibodies are available commercially now. Some people do not produce heterophile antibodies in response to EBV infection, so serological tests measuring antibodies to viral proteins, viral capsid antigen (VCA), EBV early antigen (EBV-EA), and EBV nuclear antigens (EBNA) have been developed.

Influenza viruses affect respiratory epithelial cells and become established there, with respiratory secretion being the transmission mode. Symptoms in adults include fever, headache, photophobia, sore muscles, malaise, and a sore throat. Once again, CD8+ T cells and natural killer cells are the main effector cells in the elimination of the influenza virus, as they kill virally infected cells. B cells neutralize the virus and prevent attachment and entry into cells. Antibodies are made to both HA and NA antigens.

Phagocytes will endocytose influenza virus, with or without opsonins, when the virus is outside the cell. Influenza virus inhibits lysosomal fusion with phagosomes however, and hampers the cytotoxic capability of the phagocyte. Without lysosomal enzymes in the phagosome, microbial destruction requires nitric oxide production. There are many types of influenza vaccines developed mostly with whole, inactivated viruses or split/subunit virions, but immunological responses and protection are often inadequate. New adjuvants and genetically engineered vaccines are therefore being developed. Two tests used to detect influenza antigens in clinical samples are the endogenous viral encoded enzyme assay and an optical immunoassay, although tests can be used to detect the presence of influenza virus or antibodies in clinical specimens as well.

Human polioviruses (types 1, 2, and 3) are in salivary and respiratory droplets, as well as in feces. Infection starts with attachment to a specific cellular receptor, and internalization into cells of the oropharynx. Some virions spread to the tonsils, others go into the saliva and pass into the digestive tract. Polioviruses have a tropism for epithelial cells of the intestine, in which some released virions are shed into fecal secretions where they are contagious. Infections may be asymptomatic or present as mild flu-like illnesses with fever, myalgia, nausea, gastrointestinal disturbances, and sore throat. Rarely, the virus spreads to the spinal cord, and/or brain stem where it infects and damages cells of the nervous system.

Three factors contribute to the outcome of polio virus infection: virulence of the poliovirus strain, number of infecting virions, and immunological status of the individual. As with other viral infections, CD8+ T cells and natural killer cells play major roles in resolution of the infection, and IgM, IgG, and IgA antibodies are made.

Immunization with inactivated or attenuated poliovirus is part of the recommended immunization schedule, and two types of polio vaccines are currently licensed in North America: the Salk vaccine and the Oral Sabin vaccine. The Salk vaccine is a mixture of three serotypes inactivated, whereas the Sabin-type attenuated oral poliovirus vaccine is available in two forms, trivalent and monovalent. Polio cases are rare in countries where the polio vaccine is part of the recommended immunization schedule, and in those infrequent cases, virus may be isolated from a throat swab, saliva, and nasal secretions prior to symptoms and for a few days after the illness has developed. After that, the virus may be detected in feces. Serological tests have limited value since there are many serotypes, so serology is used to confirm that the isolated virus in the clinical specimen was triggering an immune response and was not simply a passenger virus not contributing to the disease process.

REVIEW OF KEY TERMS AND ABBREVIATIONS

Matching: Match the key term in the left column with the definition in the right column.

Matching: Match the key term in the left column with the definition in the right column.

1. _____ acute phase

a) virus is diminishing during this period of the disease

2. _____ adenoids

b) cytokines released from virally infected cells

3. _____ adenovirus

c) minor mutations in HA and NA

4. _____ adjuvant

d) member of *herpesviridae* with double stranded DNA

5. _____ antigenic drifts

e) lymph nodules found in the ileum

6. _____ antigenic shifts

f) added to vaccine to enhance immune response

7. _____ asymptomatic

g) normal heterophile antibodies found in sera of most normal individuals

8. _____ convalescent phase

h) glycoprotein in influenza virus required for cell entry

9. _____ cytomegalovirus

i) able to fight off disease and infection

10. _____ Epstein Barr virus

j) lymphatic tissue in the recess of the nasopharynx

11. _____ fluad

k) single stranded segmented RNA enveloped virus

12. _____ Forssman antibodies

l) antibodies made to antigen in one species, cross reactive

13. _____ glycophorin

m) major changes in HA and NA

14. _____ HA

n) endogenous enzyme on surface of influenza A and B

15. _____ heterophile

o) free of signs and symptoms of disease or infection

16. _____ immunocompetent

p) red blood cell antigen

17. _____ IM

q) virus is fully active during this period of disease

18. _____ influenza virus

r) influenza vaccine

19. _____ interferons

s) member of *herpesviridae* with double stranded DNA

20. _____ neuraminidase

    t) infects lymphoid tissues; Epstein Barr virus is cause

21. _____ Peyer's patches

    u) common *adenoviridae* family pathogen; naked DNA

Definitions: Write the definition of each of the following words or terms.

1. acute phase _____

_____

2. adenoids _____

_____

3. adenovirus _____

_____

4. adjuvant _____

_____

5. antigenic drift _____

_____

6. antigenic shift _____

_____

7. cytomegalovirus _____

_____

8. asymptomatic _____

_____

9. Epstein Barr virus _____

_____

10. convalescent phase _____

_____

11. immunocompetent _____

_____

12. infectious mononucleosis _____

_____

13. poliovirus _____

_____

REVIEW EXERCISES

True or False: Read each statement and decide if it is TRUE or FALSE. Place T or F on the line before each statement.

1. _____ Adenovirus is an enveloped RNA virus first isolated from adenoids.

2. _____ Most adenoviral infections are symptomatic.

3. _____ The most common route for adenoviral infection is the respiratory tract.

4. _____ CMV infections are a major cause of mortality in the immunosuppressed.

5. _____ CytoGam is IV solution of gamma globulins with anti-CMV antibodies.

Fill in the Blank: Complete the following sentences on the immune system by filling in the missing word or words.

1. The adenovirus was first isolated from _____ .

2. Entry of naked virions into cells is poorly understood, however _____ following receptor binding is the most likely mechanism.

3. The adenovirus is used as a _____ in gene therapy.

4. _____ is the virus most frequently transmitted *in utero*.

5. _____ is an intravenous solution of gamma globulins.

Multiple Choice: Choose the best answer.

1. The fact that CMV infections manifest primarily in the immunosuppressed or neonates emphasizes the role of _____ in immune surveillance.

   a. macrophages
   b. class I MHC-viral peptide
   c. gamma globulins
   d. B cells
   e. T cells

2. Substances added to a vaccine to enhance immune response for higher antibody titer are

   a. antibodies.
   b. gamma globulins.
   c. opsonins.
   d. adjuvants like alum formulation or MF59.
   e. fluorescent molecules.

3. Used to detect CMV nucleic acids in a fixed clinical sample.

   a. assays that use amplification techniques
   b. *in situ* hybridization
   c. latex agglutination
   d. complement fixation
   e. PCR

4. Addresses problem of latent or active infection of CMV.

   a. detect CMV mRNA within host cells
   b. detect CMV DNA in peripheral blood cells
   c. hybrid capture technique
   d. chemiluminescence
   e. labeled anti-hybrid antibodies

CRITICAL THINKING EXERCISE

You have just started microbiology class this morning and all your classmates are introducing themselves. Most all the students in class are either in nursing or medical technology except the student sitting right next to you. Her name is Tamara, and she is interested in the dental hygiene program. Tamara also announces to the class by way of introduction that she has just gotten over infectious mononucleosis (IM). You are visibly alarmed, but your instructor says that the virus causing IM is infectious but not highly contagious.

1. What virus causes IM? What does your instructor mean by this virus being infectious but not very contagious? Does that comfort you? Why or why not?

2. How is the virus transmitted, and what is its primary cell target? How did this virus receive its name, and what other infections or diseases are associated with it?

3. How do acute clinical diseases of this virus manifest? How does this virus behave in the body over time? What evasive strategies has this virus evolved to thwart the immune system? Why is anemia associated with IM?

4. What are heterophile antibodies, and how is their routine detection associated with diagnosis of IM? What immunizations are available for this virus, and what is one of the problems with the vaccines?

5. Describe some laboratory diagnoses of the virus that causes IM.

RETROVIRAL INFECTIONS

OUTLINE

OBJECTIVES

Upon completion of this chapter, the reader should be able to:

1. Provide a brief description of the human acquired immunodeficiency virus, the causative agent of acquired immunodeficiency syndrome.
2. Briefly describe the clinical manifestations of HIV infections.
3. Explain the role of the immune system and the effectors in host defense as a response to infections with HIV.
4. Discuss the availability of vaccines, or the status of vaccine development, for HIV.
5. Describe the serological laboratory tests that are available for diagnosis of HIV.

SUMMARY OF KEY POINTS

Retroviruses have an RNA genome, which must be converted to double stranded DNA after entry into a host cell; this requires the concerted action of three enzymes: viral protease (cleaves and activates reverse transcriptase), reverse transcriptase (mediates conversion of RNA to DNA), and integrase (integrates DNA into the host genome). The integrated viral DNA is referred to as a provirus, which may be silent or actively transcribed into the RNA genome and mRNA, then translated to viral proteins with assembly occurring at the cell surface where the retroviruses acquire an envelope as they bud from the cell.

Human immunodeficiency viruses type 1 and type 2 (HIV-1 and HIV-2) cause progressive loss of immune system function. Protruding from the lipid envelope is the gp120/gp41 protein complex. The main receptor for CD4 molecules on T cells, dendritic cells like Langerhans cells, and macrophages, is the gp120 molecule. A co-receptor is requisite for infection as well: a chemokine receptor (CCR5 or CXCR4).

Detectable anti-HIV antibodies (seroconversion) are apparent within a month, but detection may not be possible for three to six months. Manifestations of HIV infection are asymptomatic to development of opportunistic infections, cancer, and loss of immune system function altogether, referred to as acquired immunodeficiency syndrome (AIDS). HIV transmission occurs via routes such as sexual contact, blood or blood product transfusion, needle sharing, and transplantation of tissues or organs. Most common transmission is through vaginal infection during unprotected intercourse. Transmission may be made from mother to child during pregnancy or breast-feeding, and accounts for about seven percent of HIV infection worldwide. HIV-1 and HIV-2 are very similar in morphology and infectivity, and several strains of HIV-1 have been isolated.

Immunological aberrations as a consequence of these infections include a decrease in number of CD4+ T cells, hypergammaglobulinemia (increased level of circulating antibodies), and a decreased capacity for phagocytosis. As CD4+ T cells produce cytokines required for all aspects of the immune system, the effect of a decreasing CD4+ T cell population has disastrous consequences.

More than 30 candidate HIV vaccines have been investigated, but they have not provided both humoral and cellular host immunity. A prime boost approach consisting of a DNA plasmid (injected intradermally with a gene gun or intramuscularly with a syringe) and a boost component of an attenuated vaccinia virus with HIV genes shows promise however.

A two-step approach is used to diagnose HIV in the laboratory where first the patient sample is screened using an enzyme immunoassay (e.g., ELISA). Positive and equivocal samples are then tested using a western blot approach. New approaches measure the viral load in serum, and some assays are based on amplification of viral nucleic acid or focus on signal amplification. Three amplification assays widely tested are the Amplicor HIV-1 Monitor (Roche Diagnostics), HIV-1 RNA (Bayer), and HIV-1 QT RNA (Organon Tecknika).

Human T cell leukemia viruses (HTLV) are members of the *Retroviridae* family, and three types have been identified: HTLV-1, HTLV-2, and HTLV-5 associated with different diseases. HTLV-1 has been most extensively studied, and is associated with adult T cell leukemia (ATL). Transmitted through sexual contact, contaminated blood or blood products, as well from mother to child through breast milk, most individuals with HTLV-1 are asymptomatic with long incubation periods before symptoms might manifest in lymphocytosis (increase in white blood cells), which is sometimes called pre-adult T cell leukemia.

Less than five percent of infected individuals develop adult T cell leukemia (ATL), and very small percent (1–3%) may develop tropical spastic paralysis (TSP) also called HTLV-1 associated myelopathy (HAM). TSP or HAM is characterized by spinal cord inflammation leading to progressive weakness in the legs. HTLV-1 can be isolated from cerebral spinal fluid as well as from serum in these patients with TSP.

The infected cell rather than the virion is the most significant immunological target for host defense, since the HTLV infects cells where it is sequestered from host defenses. High serum levels of IgM are associated with patients with HTLV-1 infection who develop HAM/TSP, suggesting the viral antigens are continuously being released into circulation or that some T cell defect has occurred hindering iso-type switching. Increased levels of Type 1 cytokines cause inflammation in these patients, and cytotoxic T cells can be found from the blood and cerebral spinal fluid. Since T cells proliferate in the absence of a triggering signal, dysregulation of the immune response in HTLV-1 infection is obvious, so that the number of CD8+ T cells is excessively enhanced.

There is no vaccine for protection from HTLV, though investigations focus on animal models to develop vaccine strategies to elicit protective immunity. Indirect immunofluorescence and particle ag-glutination tests are commercially available.

REVIEW OF KEY TERMS AND ABBREVIATIONS

Matching: Match the key term in the left column with the definition in the right column.

1. _____ acid citrate dextrose

2. _____ AIDS

3. _____ amplicor

4. _____ HIV

5. _____ hypergammaglobulinemia

6. _____ Langerhans cells

7. _____ MVA

8. _____ prime-boost

9. _____ proviral DNA

10. _____ provirus

11. _____ retrovirus

12. _____ reverse transcriptase

13. _____ Ru probe

14. _____ TMB

15. _____ TSP

16. _____ viral protease

a) assay to measure HIV-1 in plasma

b) integrated viral RNA; proviral DNA

c) alpha, beta, delta cells in pancreas

d) a viral enzyme

e) viral genes excised and HIV genes inserted

f) integrated viral RNA; provirus

g) HTLV-1 associated myelopathy (HAM)

h) an anticoagulant

i) enveloped single stranded RNA viruses

j) increased level of circulating antibodies

k) a viral enzyme

l) member of *Retroviridae*; loss of immune system

m) horseradish peroxidase substrate

n) DNA vaccine later to enhance primary vaccine

o) Ruthenium

p) total breakdown of immune system

Definitions: Write the definition of each of the following words or terms.

1. acid citrate dextrose _____

    _____

2. acquired immunodeficiency syndrome _____

    _____

3. amplicor HIV monitor test _____

    _____

4. antibody capture _____

    _____

5. human immunodeficiency virus _____

    _____

6. human T cell leukemia viruses _____

    _____

7. hypergammaglobulinemia _____

    _____

8. Langerhans cells _____

    _____

9. modified vaccinia ankara-strain _____

    _____

10. prime-boost _____

    _____

11. provirus _____

    _____

12. retroviruses _____

    _____

13. tropical spastic paraparesis _____

    _____

REVIEW EXERCISES

True or False: Read each statement and decide if it is TRUE or FALSE. Place T or F on the line before each statement.

1. _____ Retroviruses have RNA genomes converted to double stranded DNA.

2. _____ CD4 is necessary, but not sufficient for HIV entry into host cells.

3. _____ All HIV infected cells have CD4 protein on their surface.

4. _____ Viral RNA can be detected using nucleic acid amplification techniques.

5. _____ B cell activation and differentiation follow HIV infection.

Fill in the Blank: Complete the following sentences on the immune system by filling in the missing word or words.

1. _____ are enveloped, single stranded RNA viruses whose RNA genome is converted to double stranded DNA following entry into a host cell.

2. _____ are the three enzymes contained within the HIV capsid.

3. Released infectious particles are referred to as _____ .

4. Integrated viral RNA is referred to as _____ .

5. Most documented cases of _____ have been associated with HIV-1 infection.

Multiple Choice: Choose the best answer.

1. Infected _____ have been isolated from both the female vagina and male foreskin epithelia.

   a. macrophages
   b. T cells
   c. B cells
   d. M cells
   e. Langerhans cells

2. Attachment of HIV is mediated by the interaction of the _____ with CD4.

   a. gp41
   b. p17
   c. p24
   d. gp120
   e. CCR5

3. Chemokine receptors, CCR5 and CXCR4, are referred to as co-receptors and induce changes in _____ resulting in the fusion of the viral particle with the host cell membrane followed by viral entry into cell.

   a. gp120
   b. gp41
   c. CD4
   d. CD8
   e. p17

4. Coverts viral RNA to double stranded DNA.

   a. reverse transcriptase
   b. integrase
   c. protease
   d. CCR5
   e. CD4

CRITICAL THINKING EXERCISE

Your wife, who is a nursing student, has just spent an entire summer in Zambia, Zimbabwe, and Rwanda. While she was there, she was most definitely working with individuals with AIDS and working closely with the people who were most ill. Of course, she took universal precautions as all the nursing and clinical staff did. Your wife returns to tell you that many individuals are known there who repeatedly are directly exposed to HIV and do not seroconvert and seem to remain unaffected, and also that there is much controversy and debate in the countries of Africa over circumcision as some prevention of HIV infection.

1. What is seroconversion? How do you and your wife explain how individuals can be exposed to HIV, but apparently not become infected?

2. How might circumcision be related to HIV infection or not?

3. What immunological aberrations manifest as a consequence of HIV infection?

4. What immunization approaches have been investigated for HIV vaccines?

5. Cite laboratory diagnostic techniques used for HIV.

CHAPTER 23

FUNGAL INFECTIONS

OUTLINE

- *Aspergillus fumigatus*
  - Clinical Manifestations/Pathology
  - Immunology
  - Immunization Progress
  - Laboratory Diagnosis
- *Candida albicans*
  - General Features
  - Clinical Manifestations/Pathology
  - Immunology
  - Immunization
  - Laboratory Diagnosis
- *Cryptococcus neoformans*
  - Clinical Manifestations/Pathology
  - Immunology
  - Immunization Progress
  - Laboratory Diagnosis

OBJECTIVES

Upon completion of this chapter, the reader should be able to:

1. Provide a brief description of the opportunistic fungi that cause mycotic infections.
2. Briefly describe the clinical manifestations of mycotic infections caused by the opportunistic fungi *Aspergillus fumigatus*, *Candida albicans*, and *Cryptococcus neoformans*.

3. Explain the role of the immune system and the effectors in host defense to the opportunistic fungi *Aspergillus fumigatus*, *Candida albicans*, and *Cryptococcus neoformans*. As well, the reader should be able to describe the evasive strategies employed to establish infection.

4. Discuss the availability of vaccines, or the status of vaccine development to control infections with *Aspergillus fumigatus*, *Candida albicans*, and *Cryptococcus neoformans*.

5. Describe the current laboratory tests that are available for diagnosis of each of these opportunistic fungi.

SUMMARY OF KEY POINTS

Aspergillus spp., ubiquitous fungi, are opportunistic, and infections with members of this genus are called aspergillosis. Diseases range from superficial or noninvasive in the immunocompetent to allergic aspergillosis, and even invasive infection in immunocompromised hosts. *Aspergillus fumigatus* is the most commonly infectious species in humans. Allergic bronchopulmonary aspergillosis, referred to as farmer's lung, occurs when a substantial number of airborne spores are inhaled.

Phagocytes are the first-line defense for *Aspergillus spp.* infections, and phagocyte cytotoxic function is enhanced by Type 1 cytokines, a sufficient amount of Type 1 cytokine being required early in the immune response for effective host defense. No vaccine is available for *Aspergillus spp.*, and diagnosis is difficult with antigen detection usually requiring invasive biopsy. Commercial latex agglutination tests for the detection of serum *Aspergillus* polysaccharide (galactomannan) antigens as well as an immunoenzymatic sandwich microplate technique are available. Immunodiffusion is the most widely used technique for antibody detection commercially available.

Candida albicans is part of the normal flora, competing with other resident bacteria for an ecological niche in mucous membranes, especially in the gastrointestinal tract; but *Candida albicans* is controlled by the immune system and by environmental factors, most notably pH. Like *Aspergillus*, *C. albicans* is an opportunistic fungus, becoming pathogenic only when an individual is immunosuppressed. Superficial skin or mucous infections all the way to systemic infection of organs is possible, with mucocutaneous or deep tissue infection by *C. albicans* referred to as Candidiasis. *C. albicans* has a number of polysaccharides such as glucan, chitin, and mannan on its cell surface, which are often covalently linked to proteins forming mannoproteins. These mannoproteins are the major antigenic determinants for Candida, and are important for development of vaccines and laboratory analysis. *C. albicans* are yeast-like with asexual reproduction occurring by the multilateral production of blastoconidia (buds) extending out from the cell. Pseudohyphae are made when the buds form one after the other in a linear fashion, with the pseudohyphae looking like sausage links attached to the main body.

No vaccine for Candida is available for humans, but animal studies have demonstrated protective immunity from immunization. Test kits for easy detection of cultured colonies, and rapid point-of-care tests detecting *C. albicans* in a vaginal smear are available commercially.

Cryptococcus neoformans, found in soil and avian droppings, is an encapsulated, yeast-like fungus causing systemic disease in humans. *C. neoformans* is not found in fresh droppings, but rather droppings from sites like window ledges where in a dry environment it becomes encapsulated and reduced in size. Airborne, *C. neoformans* can be inhaled and invade the lungs, where it becomes hydrated and acquires its polysaccharide capsule.

Headache, optic neuritis, fever, and seizures are manifestations of a *C. neoformans* infection. Individuals with T cell immunodeficiencies are at highest risk of *C. neoformans* infection. Virulence of *C. neoformans* is derived in large measure from the protection it receives from its polysaccharide capsule, which prevents its non-opsonin-mediated phagocytosis. Also, *C. neoformans* secretes substances hindering its destruction in the phagocytic vacuole. Effector molecules secreted by activated B cells and CD4+

T cells of the adaptive immune system can override these *C. neoformans* protective mechanisms however. B cells through their differentiated plasma cells form and secrete antibodies, and T cells secrete cytokines.

A phase 1 clinical trial is being done to determine safety and immunogenicity of a *C. neoformans* polysaccharide-tetanus toxoid vaccine conjugate in human subjects. Test kits are available to aid in diagnosis of *C. neoformans*; some are designed to detect anti-*C. neoformans* antibodies while others test for the C. neoformans antigens.

REVIEW OF KEY TERMS AND ABBREVIATIONS

Matching: Match the key term in the left column with the definition in the right column.

1. _____ aflatoxin

a) airborne particles from *Aspergillus spp.*

2. _____ asexual

b) solid phase sandwich detects galactomannan

3. _____ aspergillosis

c) rapid point-of-care test for C. polysaccharide

4. _____ spores

d) activation of NADPH oxidase enzyme complex

5. _____ CAND-TEC

e) when inducible nitric oxide synthase is activated

6. _____ chromogenic medium

f) thick yellow or milky discharge clinically

7. _____ crypto-LA test

g) made when *Aspergillus* grows on wheat, peanuts

8. _____ Farmer's lung

h) specimen is cultured 48 hours at RT for five days

9. _____ fungal balls

i) microorganisms naturally present in environment

10. _____ intranasal

j) culture allows differential isolation *Candida spp.*

11. _____ murex test

k) white cheesy plaque on mucosal surface

12. _____ nitric oxide

l) mycetomas

13. _____ normal flora

m) simple rapid test detects *C. albicans*

14. _____ opportunistic

n) invasive pulmonary infection; *Aspergillus*-caused

15. _____ oricult-N system

o) allergic infection, *Aspergillus* spores inhaled

16. _____ pastorex *Aspergillus*

p) organisms cause disease in immunocompromised

17. _____ platelia *Aspergillus*

q) single latex agglutination test with rabbit antibodies

18. _____ QUIK-TRI/CAN

    r) latex agglutination detects *Aspergillus* in serum

19. _____ thrush

    s) detects polysaccharide antigen of *C. neoformans*

20. _____ reactive oxygen intermediates

    t) through the nostril and nasal passages

21. _____ vaginal candidiasis

    u) without male and female reproductive organs

Definitions: Write the definition of each of the following words or terms.

1. aflatoxin _____

_____

2. asexual _____

_____

3. aspergillosis _____

_____

4. *Aspergillus* spores _____

_____

5. *Candida albicans* _____

_____

6. *Cryptococcus neoformans* _____

_____

7. mucocutaneous candidiasis _____

_____

8. thrush _____

_____

9. vaginal candidiasis _____

_____

10. opportunistic fungi _____

_____

11. normal flora _____

_____

12. nitric oxide _____

_____

13. murex *Cryptococcus* test _____

_____

REVIEW EXERCISES

True or False: Read each statement and decide if it is TRUE or FALSE. Place T or F on the line before each statement.

1. _____   Aspergillosis is an invasive pulmonary infection caused by *Aspergillus*.

2. _____   *Aspergillus flavus* produces a toxin, aflatoxin, when growing on peanuts.

3. _____   Complement fixation may detect anti-*Aspergillus* antibodies.

4. _____   *Candida* species are not often part of the normal flora.

5. _____   Blastoconidia (buds) form one after another making pseudohyphae.

Fill in the Blank: Complete the following sentences on the immune system by filling in the missing word or words.

1. _____ is an invasive pulmonary infection and disseminated disease caused by members of the genus *Aspergillus*.

2. *Aspergillus spp.* are _____ in that they cause disease primarily in immunosuppressed hosts.

3. Some species of *Aspergillus* (*A. flavus*) produce a toxin, a _____ , when they grow on wheat, peanuts, or rice.

4. Presence of *Aspergillus spp.* in the _____ host does not cause invasive disease, however chronic sinus infection and allergic aspergillosis may occur.

5. _____ may develop in pulmonary cavities secondary to tuberculosis disease following inhalation of *Aspergillus* spores.

Multiple Choice: Choose the best answer.

1. Almost every aspect of immunity is regulated by

   a. cytokines.
   b. chemokines.
   c. B cells.
   d. T cells.
   e. phagocytes.

2. Latex agglutination test for detection of serum Aspergillus polysaccharide (galactomannan) commercially available.

   a. platelia *Aspergillus*
   b. pastorex *Aspergillus*
   c. ELISA
   d. complement fixation
   e. murex

3. Commonly used test to screen for the presence of anti-*Aspergillus* antibodies in patient sera is the double immunodiffusion test, more commonly referred to as the

   a. Ouchterlony method.
   b. Pastorex.
   c. Platelia.
   d. solid phase sandwich technique.
   e. complement fixation.

4. The major antigenic determinants for *Candida* are

   a. glucan.
   b. chitin.
   c. mannan.
   d. mannoproteins.
   e. mannose.

CRITICAL THINKING EXERCISE

Theresa, an elderly woman who is bed-ridden, has an in-dwelling catheter. Her past medical history reveals vaginal candidiasis and thrush following a prolonged antibiotic therapy. Additionally, she is at high risk for decubitus ulcers because she is bed-ridden.

1. Since *Candida albicans* has been a part of her medical history, what health areas are of major concern in her present state? What is the *Candida* connection to prolonged antibiotic therapy? an in-dwelling catheter? decubitus ulcers?

2. What clinical manifestations might one expect from *Candida* infections? What environmental factors control *Candida*? What two sites does the immune system control *Candida* infections?

3. Morphologically altered forms of *Candida* present special challenges to the immune system. How? What is the chief danger to Theresa posed by *Candida*?

4. What vaccine delivery strategies for *C. albicans* have been investigated using animal models?

5. Describe laboratory diagnosis of *C. albicans*.

CHAPTER 24

PARASITIC INFECTIONS

OUTLINE

- Amebic Infections
  - Clinical Manifestations/Pathology
  - Immunology
  - Immunization Progress
  - Laboratory Diagnosis
- Echinococcosis: *Echinococcus granulosus*
  - Definitive
  - Intermediate Hosts
  - Definitive Hosts
  - Clinical Manifestations/Pathology
  - Immunology
  - Immunization Progress
  - Laboratory Diagnosis
- Malaria
  - Life Cycle
  - Clinical Manifestations/Pathology
  - Immunology
  - Immunization
  - Laboratory Diagnosis
- *Toxoplasma gondii*
  - Intestinal-Epithelial Stage
  - Extra-Intestinal Stage
  - Clinical Manifestations/Pathology
  - Immunology

■ Immunization Progress

■ Laboratory Diagnosis

OBJECTIVES

Upon completion of this chapter, the reader should be able to:

1. Provide a brief description of the parasites that cause echinococcosis, amebic infections, malaria, and toxoplasmosis.

2. Briefly describe the clinical manifestations of the parasitic infections echinococcosis, amebic infections, malaria, and toxoplasmosis.

3. Explain the role of the immune system and the effectors in host defense to the following parasites: *Echinococcus granulosus, Entamoeba histolytica, Plasmodium falciparum,* and *Toxoplasma gondii.* As well, the reader should be able to describe the evasive strategies employed to establish infection.

4. Discuss the availability of vaccines, or the status of vaccine development to control infections with *Echinococcus granulosus, Entamoeba histolytica, Plasmodium falciparum,* and *Toxoplasma gondii.*

5. Describe the current laboratory tests that are available for diagnosis of *Echinococcus granulosus, Entamoeba histolytica, Plasmodium falciparum,* and *Toxoplasma gondii.*

SUMMARY OF KEY POINTS

Naegleria fowleri is a free-living ameba, causing primary amebic meningoencephalitis (in which fatality rates are greater than 95%) occurring primarily in children and young adults. *N. fowleri* can live outside a host, and is found in soil and in warm, fresh water (where they feed on bacteria).

Acanthamoeba spp. (six species are known to cause human disease) are free-living amebas found in tap water, bottled mineral water, chlorinated swimming pools, sea water, and soil. Amebic keratitis occurs in immunocompetent individuals using non-sterile solutions such as tap water or home-made saline to wash their contact lenses. Swimming in contaminated water with contact lenses presents a risk for amebic keratitis as well.

Entamoeba histolytica, a major pathogenic parasite for humans and found worldwide particularly in the tropics, has a fecal-oral transmission route. Symptoms and signs of the acute intestinal form of amebiasis include abdominal cramps, nausea, and severe diarrhea with mucus and blood in the stool. Vaccines for *E. histolytica* are still in preclinical phase, but the SREHP structural protein in a recombinant form is at present the most likely candidate; packaging and delivery methods for the vaccine are being investigated. Diagnosis of *E. histolytica* has been classically done via detection of the cyst form in feces, but more recent enzyme immunoassays and molecular-based diagnostic tests have been developed. In more developed countries, flow cytometry has been used to detect pathogenic amebas in water samples.

Echinococcosis or hydatid disease is a larval tapeworm infection caused by ingesting food contaminated with tapeworm eggs. Humans are only occasional intermediate hosts, but this can lead to serious disease in which the eggs hatch to larvae in the intestinal tract, penetrate the intestinal wall, and enter the circulation. In this extracellular stage the parasite is vulnerable to immunological host defenses. There is no vaccine for use in humans to preclude infection with *Echinococcus granulosus,* but a vaccine using recombinant *E. granulosus* proteins has been tested in sheep and induced more than 90% protection in subsequent challenge infections. Laboratory diagnosis includes ultrasound, CAT scan, or MRI imaging techniques demonstrating a cyst, with serological tests complementing the medical imaging (especially ultrasound).

Malaria is a parasitic infection caused by *Plasmodium spp.* with the definitive host being the Anopheles mosquito. Humans are intermediate hosts in which asexual forms develop. Malaria presents with abrupt fever, malaise, myalgia, and headache typically. Infection occurs when a *Plasmodium* species enters the blood stream as a motile infective sporozoite during a mosquito bite. After entering the liver, the parasite differentiates into the merozoite form and is released back into the blood stream where it enters red blood cells. While inside red blood cells the merozoite begins a cyclic differentiation stage to gametocytes or to merozoites via trophozoite and schizont intermediates. These are released into the blood stream when the red blood cell ruptures. Merozoites infect red blood cells and the cyclic process is repeated with red blood cell destruction. Gametocytes do not cause pathology, nor do they form zygotes. Zygotes are only formed if a mosquito takes up the gametocytes during a blood meal. The brief time in which the malarial parasite is outside cells (extracellular) hampers the generation of a productive immune response, and also the parasitic forms or entities in circulation differ during the course of an infection.

Several vaccines have been and are being tested, and although some have met with partial success, no single vaccine has yet been able to provide long-term immunity. There is a transmission-blocking vaccine that makes anti-zygote antibodies with the rationale that the mosquito will ingest antibodies and gametocytes. When a zygote is formed, ingested antibodies will preclude their differentiation and secretion in saliva. When there is difficulty in identifying the ring forms on blood films or in cases when the number of malarial parasites in peripheral blood is so low they escape detection on a blood slide, then there are tests to detect either anti-malarial antibodies or malaria antigens, or malarial enzymes.

Toxoplasma gondii is an intestinal parasite and the causative agent of toxoplasmosis. The cat family is the definitive host for *T. gondii*, but a number of mammals including humans may serve as intermediate hosts. Asexual reproduction occurs in intermediate hosts with sexual reproduction only occurring in the definitive host. Uncooked, infected meat (e.g., pork, sheep containing the bradyzoite form in a cyst) is the source of *T. gondii* infection in adults, or through fecal matter (oocytes). After ingestion the cyst wall is ruptured and the released bradyzoites enter epithelial cells lining the intestine. Some bradyzoites will release on the basolateral side of the epithelial cells, undergo asexual reproduction, and disseminate to other tissues. If the host is the definitive host, sexual reproduction occurs in the epithelial cells.

T. gondii infections (chronic) in healthy adults are usually asymptomatic with localized swelling of lymph nodes. Sometimes, flu-like symptoms accompany the infection. An immunocompromised individual will have widespread infection, however, and it may even become fatal. If a pregnant woman becomes infected, major developmental abnormalities may occur in the fetus (congenital toxoplasmosis), but the extent is determined by the stage of development when the mother was infected.

Resolution of *T. gondii* infection results in protective immunity. When the parasites are released from ruptured cells, they are susceptible to phagocytic action. Type 1 cytokines generated by CD4+ T cells enhance the action of the phagocyte. B cells specific for the parasite will be activated and differentiation to antibody-secreting plasma cells. Animal studies show that effective immunization may become a reality in the future. Serological testing is the main way to diagnose, but kits detecting IgM or IgG antibodies specific for *T. gondii* are commercially available.

REVIEW OF KEY TERMS AND ABBREVIATIONS

Matching: Match the key term in the left column with the definition in the right column.

1. _____ *Acanthamoeba*   a) tissue anoxia of the brain

2. _____ ameba   b) red blood cells

3. _____ amebic colitis   c) liver parenchymal cells

4. _____ cerebral malaria

    d) organism in which larvae develop into adult worms

5. _____ congenital toxoplasmosis

    e) parasitic infection caused by *Plasmodium spp.*

6. _____ cyst

    f) body temperature above normal

7. _____ definitive host

    g) an adhesion molecule

8. _____ erythrocytes

    h) do not need host for survival

9. _____ excystation

    i) organelles of movement on ameba

10. _____ fever

    j) thrive only when in a host

11. _____ free-living ameba

    k) dormant form of ameba

12. _____ gametes

    l) female merozoite

13. _____ hepatocytes

    m) free-living ameba found in environment

14. _____ hydatid cysts

    n) disease caused by *E. histolytica* in large intestine

15. _____ lectin

    o) parasite form in encapsulated nucleus

16. _____ macrogametocyte

    p) sex cells

17. _____ malaria

    q) small one-celled organism moving by pseudopods

18. _____ merozoite

    r) multinucleated form of parasite

19. _____ obligate parasites

    s) parasite escapes the cyst wall

20. _____ pseudopodia

    t) tissue growth as result of parasitic worm infection

21. _____ schizont

    u) contracted by a woman during pregnancy

Definitions: Write the definition of each of the following words or terms.

1. ameba _____

   _____

2. amebic colitis _____

   _____

3. bradyzoites _____

   _____

4. congenital toxoplasmosis _____

_____

5. definitive host _____

_____

6. Echinococcosis _____

_____

7. erythrocytes _____

_____

8. hepatocytes _____

_____

9. hydatid cysts _____

_____

10. intermediate host _____

_____

11. merozoite microgametocyte _____

_____

12. protoscoleces _____

_____

13. zygote _____

_____

REVIEW EXERCISES

True or False: Read each statement and decide if it is TRUE or FALSE. Place T or F on the line before each statement.

1. _____   There are no free-living amebas.

2. _____   Amebas are typically found as feeding trophozoites or dormant cysts.

3. _____   Bottled water should be considered free of parasites.

4. _____   Primary amebic meningoencephalitis has fatality rates greater than 95%!

5. _____   Most cases of *E. histolytica* infections are in third world countries.

Fill in the Blank: Complete the following sentences on the immune system by filling in the missing word or words.

1. Amebas exist either as _____ that thrive only when in a host, or as free-living amebas that exist primarily in the environment.

2. Motility of the trophozoite is achieved by extensions of _____ .

3. _____ are free-living amebas found throughout the environment.

4. Local tissue damage, multinucleated giant cells, and lots of activated mononuclear phagocytes characterize _____ .

5. _____ occurs in immunocompetent individuals that have used non-sterile solutions such as tap water or home-made saline to wash their contact lenses.

Multiple Choice: Choose the best answer.

1. All of the following are clinical manifestations during infection of the brain except

   a. nausea.
   b. vomiting.
   c. seizures.
   d. altered mental states.
   e. keratitis.

2. Patients with this report photophobia.

   a. amebic keratitis
   b. pneumonitis
   c. dermatitis
   d. sinusitis
   e. immunosuppression

3. *Naegleria fowleri* causes this disease with 95% fatality rates or greater.

   a. granulomatous amebic encephalitis
   b. primary amebic meningoencephalitis
   c. amebic colitis
   d. hydatid cysts
   e. toxoplasmosis

4. Parasitic infection caused by _____ *spp.* results in malaria.

   a. *Toxoplasma*
   b. *Echinococcus*
   c. *Naegleria*
   d. *Plasmodium*
   e. *Entamoeba*

CRITICAL THINKING EXERCISE

Critical Thinking/Case Study

You have a friend named Alex who is an entomologist especially interested in insects as disease vectors. Since you have read Chapter 24, you have a lot to discuss with Alex concerning malaria.

1. What is the definitive host for all the infecting *Plasmodium spp.*? What does that mean? What does Alex suggest about the life cycle of the *Plasmodium*, and how having two sorts of hosts might benefit the organism? What sorts of controls might Alex suggest?

2. What is sickle cell anemia, and what "ironic" benefit does it confer to a sufferer? What conclusions may be drawn about sickle cell anemia and malaria?

3. The life cycle of the malaria parasite is quite complex. Why is a basic understanding of it necessary before considering immunology or vaccine development? Cite the most salient features of the cycle. (Consider sporozoite and merozoite antigenic epitopes in repeat infections.)

4. What is malarial pigment? What are typical clinical manifestations and pathology of infection with *Plasmodium spp.*? In areas where malaria is endemic the incidence and severity decreases with age. Why?

5. What are the challenges for developing an effective vaccine for malaria?

6. Discuss laboratory diagnosis of malaria.

CHAPTER 25

AUTOIMMUNE DISORDERS

OUTLINE

OBJECTIVES

Upon completion of this chapter, the reader should be able to:

1. Explain what is meant by "loss of tolerance" and how this relates to autoimmune disorders.

2. Describe the general characteristics and clinical manifestations of the following autoimmune disorders: Type 1 diabetes, rheumatoid arthritis, systemic lupus erythematosus, Graves' Disease, Hashimoto's thyroiditis, and pernicious anemia.

3. Describe how the immune system contributes to the pathology of autoimmune disorders: Type 1 diabetes, rheumatoid arthritis, systemic lupus erythematosus, Graves' Disease, Hashimoto's thyroiditis, and pernicious anemia.

4. List the antigens to which specific autoantibodies are generated for each of the autoimmune disorders: Type 1 diabetes, rheumatoid arthritis, systemic lupus erythematosus, Graves' Disease, Hashimoto's thyroiditis, and pernicious anemia.

5. Explain the role of serological tests in each of the following autoimmune disorders: Type 1 diabetes, rheumatoid arthritis, systemic lupus erythematosus, Graves' Disease, Hashimoto's thyroiditis, and pernicious anemia.

SUMMARY OF KEY POINTS

The fact that the immune system is not activated when it meets its own antigens is called *self tolerance*, and autoimmunity results when there is a breakdown in self tolerance. Type 1 *diabetes mellitus* or juvenile diabetes is a chronic disorder of glucose metabolism in which there is selective destruction of the insulin-producing beta cells in the pancreatic islets. While the initiating stimulus is unknown, there are anti-insulin and anti-GAD autoantibodies present in individuals affected.

Rheumatoid arthritis is a chronic systemic inflammatory disorder whose etiology is unknown, with principal manifestations being joint pain affecting many joints simultaneously. The production of rheumatoid factor made up of IgM and IgG antibodies specific for the Fc region of IgG antibodies is associated with rheumatoid arthritis, and immune complexes (IgM-IgG; IgG-IgG) are believed to generate processes responsible for the joint inflammation (a characteristic of this autoimmune disease). Also, cytokines (e.g., IFNγ and TNF) enhance this inflammation. Tissue macrophages respond to the cytokines becoming transiently activated; activated B cells are present in the synovium but the specificity of these B cells is not known. Normal regulatory mechanisms cannot control the magnitude of the inflammatory response. Type 2 cytokines, made by CD4+ T cells, and tissue inhibitors of metalloproteinases (TIMP), made by macrophages, cannot control the response because the antigen is always present and not removed. Ongoing clinical trials are based on the principle that TNF is a major contributing factor in the pathogenesis, so anti-TNF antibodies are administered to clean up the TNF, so it may not be available to perpetuate or enhance the inflammatory response.

Another autoimmune disorder is *systemic lupus erythematosus* (SLE), characterized by the production of autoantibodies and inflammation in multiple organs including kidney and brain. In the active phase of the disease, patients experience fatigue, fever, and weight loss with clinical manifestations including skin rashes, arthritis, glomerulonephritis (kidney inflammation), anemia, thrombosis, and central nervous system involvement (headaches, seizures, or psychoses). A classic butterfly rash extends across the nose to the cheeks in about 40% of patients. In SLE, the autoantibodies target dsDNA (double-stranded DNA), where dsDNA is released into circulation when cells are damaged. Interaction of dsDNA with antibodies specific for this antigen results in complexes, which form large aggregates that may lodge in small vesicles or basement membranes. An anti-phospholipid antibody is also formed during SLE, and it is called *lupus anti-coagulant*. If anti-phospholipid antibodies cross the placenta, they may cause a spontaneous abortion. Immune complex formations do not cease unless SLE is in remission. Normal clearance mechanisms like phagocytes are unable to eliminate the large numbers of immune complexes, and the immune complexes deposit in capillary walls where they are targets for complement activation. The site of immune complex deposition determines pathology of SLE.

Graves' disease is an autoimmune disease in which the thyroid gland secretes more T3 and T4 than the body needs, and this results in enhanced metabolic activity leading to an increase in pulse rate, heat intolerance, sporadic episodes of heart palpitation, exophthalmos (bulging eyeballs), weight loss, and hair loss. Enlarged thyroid gland (goiter) is another characteristic of Graves' disease, and individuals with Graves' disease have elevated circulating levels of the thyroid hormones T3 and T4 because autoantibodies bind to TSH receptors, which stimulate unregulated secretion of these hormones. Physical examination and measurements of serum thyroid hormones T3, T4, and TSH are used to diagnose and support diagnosis respectively. In Graves' disease, T3 and T4 serum levels will be elevated while TSH levels will be low.

Hashimoto's thyroiditis is an autoimmune disease resulting in hypothyroidism, in which serum levels of T3 and T4 are decreased because cells of the immune system attack the thyroid gland. Feedback mechanisms result in an increase in TSH as the body attempts to increase T3 and T4 levels. Early on in the disease, levels of T4 and TSH are normal, but a higher titer of anti-thyroid peroxidase is observed. Later, levels of T4 decrease and levels of TSH increase.

Pernicious anemia is due to malabsorption of vitamin B12, because intrinsic factor from parietal cells of the stomach is not available to complex vitamin B12 (and transport of vitamin B12 from the gut to the blood stream is contingent on the formation of this complex). If parietal cells are destroyed or if autoantibodies (anti-intrinsic factor) bind to the intrinsic factor, then intrinsic factor is not available. Deficiency in vitamin B12 leads to impairment in the ability of the red blood cell to mature and develop normally leading to a reduction in red blood cell number and anemia.

REVIEW OF KEY TERMS AND ABBREVIATIONS

Matching: Match the key term in the left column with the definition in the right column.

1. _____ ENA

2. _____ autoantibody

3. _____ autoantigen

a) autoantibodies stimulate thyroid gland

b) pancreatic hormone essential to cellular use of glucose

c) autoimmune disease, disorder of glucose metabolism

4. ____ butterfly rash

    d) immunological non-responsiveness to self antigens

5. ____ clinical trials

    e) antibody specific for self protein

6. ____ diabetes mellitus

    f) excess activity of the thyroid

7. ____ free T4

    g) for vitamin B12 transport from intestine to blood

8. ____ GAD

    h) characteristic facial mark of SLE

9. ____ Graves' disease

    i) IgM and IgG bind to Fc region of IgG antibodies

10. ____ Hashimoto's thyroiditis

    j) fluid within joints

11. ____ hyperthyroidism

    k) manifests as severe chronic gastritis

12. ____ hypothyroidism

    l) B12 deficiency is absorption or dietary deficiency

13. ____ insulin

    m) stimulates production of antibodies in an individual

14. ____ intrinsic factor

    n) idiopathic chronic systemic inflammatory disorder

15. ____ parietal cells

    o) autoimmune disorder, hypothyroidism

16. ____ pernicious anemia

    p) tests to determine actual outcomes of hypothesis

17. ____ rheumatoid arthritis

    q) underactivity of the thyroid

18. ____ rheumatoid factor

    r) fraction of T4 not bound to protein

19. ____ Schilling test

    s) cells lining gastrointestinal tract

20. ____ self tolerance

    t) autoantibody to beta islet cell enzyme

21. ____ synovium

    u) autoantibody present in systemic lupus erythematosus

Definitions: Write the definition of each of the following words or terms.

1. anti-double stranded DNA _____

_____

2. autoantibody _____

_____

3. butterfly rash _____

_____

4. diabetes mellitus _____

_____

5. glutamic acid decarboxylase _____

_____

6. Graves' disease _____

_____

7. Hashimoto's thyroiditis _____

_____

8. insulin _____

_____

9. intrinsic factor _____

_____

10. parietal cells _____

_____

11. pernicious anemia _____

_____

12. rheumatoid arthritis _____

_____

13. synovium _____

_____

REVIEW EXERCISES

True or False: Read each statement and decide if it is TRUE or FALSE. Place T or F on the line before each statement.

1. _____   The magnitude of the inflammatory response in rheumatoid arthritis is too great for the normal negative regulatory mechanisms to be effective.

2. _____   Rheumatoid arthritis is not an autoimmune inflammatory disorder.

3. _____   Rheumatoid factor (IgM) is present in about 15% of patients with rheumatoid arthritis.

4. _____   Monoclonal antibodies could *mop up* TNF in rheumatoid arthritis.

5. _____   Rheumatoid arthritis is the most common autoimmune disorder.

Fill in the Blank: Complete the following sentences on the immune system by filling in the missing word or words.

1. In an automated system, rheumatoid factor levels are determined using _____ .

2. _____ is an autoimmune disorder characterized by the production of autoantibodies and inflammation in multiple organs.

3. Increased incidence of SLE according to ethnicity, as well as its association with inherited human leukocyte antigens (HLA), suggests an underlying _____ component to this disease.

4. A classic _____ extends across the nose to the cheeks in about 40% of patients with SLE.

5. Antibodies to _____ are present in about 65% of patients with SLE.

Multiple Choice: Choose the best answer.

1. Autoimmune disease in which autoantibodies stimulate the thyroid gland.

    a. SLE
    b. Graves' disease
    c. rheumatoid arthritis
    d. diabetes mellitus
    e. Hashimoto's thyroiditis

2. Autoimmune disease that results in hypothyroidism.

    a. SLE
    b. Graves' disease
    c. rheumatoid arthritis
    d. diabetes mellitus
    e. Hashimoto's thyroiditis

3. In Hashimoto's thyroiditis, levels of T3 and T4 are

   a. modulated.
   b. increased.
   c. decreased.
   d. not affected at all.
   e. first decreased, then increased.

4. Artifactual vesicles formed from the endoplasmic reticulum when cells are disrupted are

   a. anti-thyroglobulin.
   b. lysosomes.
   c. phagosomes.
   d. phagolysosomes.
   e. microsomes.

CRITICAL THINKING/CASE STUDY EXERCISE

In class one day your instructor describes the following symptoms: unnatural pallor, fatigue, loss of breath, lethargy, and depression. Your instructor goes on to mention possible neurological problems for this clinical situation in which the patient may experience tingling in the extremities, color blindness of blue and green, and confusion. Weight loss and a higher than usual likelihood of gastric cancer is mentioned, too.

1. What condition is your instructor probably describing? What is the connection to severe chronic gastritis?

2. What is the underlying cause of this condition? What clinical scenarios are possible?

3. What role do the parietal cells play? What tests can be performed to determine the cause of the vitamin B12 deficiency? What about anti-parietal cell antibody detection?

CHAPTER 26

TUMOR IMMUNOLOGY

OUTLINE

OBJECTIVES

Upon completion of this chapter, the reader should be able to:

1. Explain the differences between tumor specific antigens and tumor associated antigens.
2. List tumor specific antigens for various tumors.
3. Describe three tumor associated antigens and their role in monitoring various tumors.
4. Describe the role of the immune components in tumor immunology.
5. Explain how tumors may escape detection by the immune system.
6. Explain the differences between acute leukemia and chronic leukemia.
7. Explain the differences between Hodgkin's and non-Hodgkin's lymphoma.
8. List the various cell surface markers that are targeted for flow cytometric analysis to differentiate between leukemia and lymphomas arising from different cell types.
9. Describe the basic properties of multiple myeloma and the laboratory diagnosis.

SUMMARY OF KEY POINTS

Tumors are abnormal growths, which may be benign (lost growth control but surrounded by a capsule and not invasive) or malignant (lost growth control, NOT surrounded by a capsule, and have potential to invade other tissues). Tumor antigens are molecules present on the tumor cell surface, and they fall into two categories: unique tumor specific antigens (unique to the tumor) and tumor associated antigens (present on both the tumor and a limited number of normal cells, albeit at different stages of development). *De novo* expression of tumor specific antigens has several mechanisms proposed: silent gene activation leading to the synthesis of a new protein, point mutations giving rise to mutant peptides, and alteration in the structure of proteins allowing exposure of previously sequestered epitopes. Three oncofetal antigens play important roles in clinical diagnosis: alpha-fetoprotein (AFP), beta-human chorionic gonadotrophin (B-HCG), and carcinoembryonic antigen (CEA).

Investigations into tumor immunity have been complicated by the complexity of the soluble mediators and cells and integrative function and regulation of the human immune system. *In vitro* studies have been the basis for models of tumor immunology, looking at the effects of various immunological effectors such as macrophages, natural killer cells, T cells, B cells, antibodies, and complement. Classes of mechanisms proposed by which tumors may evade the immune system include: tumor antigen related, class I MHC related, and T cell related.

Two major classes of white blood cell neoproliferative disorders are leukemias and lymphomas. Leukemias arise in myeloid or lymphoid cell lineages, with some patients with both neoplasmic lineages. Lymphomas are primarily neoplasms of lymphocytes, T cells, and B cells. Plasma cell neoplasms are clones of antibody secreting cells, most commonly being multiple myeloma.

REVIEW OF KEY TERMS AND ABBREVIATIONS

Matching: Match the key term in the left column with the definition in the right column.

1. _____ 17-1A

2. _____ acute leukemia

3. _____ ALL

4. _____ AML

5. _____ AFP

6. _____ Bence Jones

7. _____ Burkitt's

8. _____ CEA

9. _____ carcinoma cells

10. _____ chronic

11. _____ lymphocytic

12. _____ CML

13. _____ libraries

14. _____ foreign

15. _____ galactin 9

16. _____ Hodgkin's

17. _____ leukemias

18. _____ lymphomas

19. _____ melanoma

20. _____ myeloid

a) sudden leukemia, short life expectancy without treatment

b) sum of all products expressed by cDNA for malignant cell

c) malignant cells of lymphoid tissue

d) Epstein Barr viral genome in all tumor cells

e) tumor cells

f) arising from B lymphocyte neoplasms

g) bone marrow cells

h) protein specific for human carcinoma cells

i) membrane protein found in serum; oncofetal antigen

j) protein for tumor specific antigens

k) from myeloid or lymphoid cell lineages

l) not originating in the body

m) more common form of leukemia with genetic component

n) uncommon, lymphoid tissue disorder

o) oncofetal antigen secreted during fetal development

p) a tumor of the skin

q) rare neoplasm increase in neutrophils and precursors

r) monoclonal proteins detected in urine

s) the malignant cell is a mature cell

t) excess proliferation of developing cell failing to mature

Definitions: Write the definition of each of the following words or terms.

1. acute leukemias _____

   _____

2. acute lymphoblastic leukemia _____

   _____

3. acute myelogenous leukemia _____

   _____

4. alpha-fetoprotein _____

   _____

5. Bence Jones proteins _____

   _____

6. beta-human chorionic gonadotrophin _____

   _____

7. Burkitt's lymphoma _____

   _____

8. carcinoembryonic antigen _____

   _____

9. chronic leukemia _____

   _____

10. tumor specific antigen _____

    _____

11. determinant selection _____

    _____

12. receptor idiotype _____

    _____

13. Philadelphia chromosome _____

    _____

REVIEW EXERCISES

True or False: Read each statement and decide if it is TRUE or FALSE. Place T or F on the line before each statement.

1. _____ T cell antigen receptors are randomly selected during T cell maturation.

2. _____ The possibility does not exist that a T cell receptor will not be formed specific for the MHC-tumor antigen peptide complexes.

3. _____ Acute leukemias involve mature cells as the malignant cell.

4. _____ A genetically altered chromosome 22 is called a Philadelphia chromosome.

5. _____ Chronic lymphocytic leukemia is usually a B cell neoplasm.

Fill in the Blank: Complete the following sentences on the immune system by filling in the missing word or words.

1. The protein _____ was shown to be present in about half of the Hodgkin's patients.

2. T cells and B cells express cell surface receptors whose variable regions or _____ are unique to a particular clone.

3. Proteins expressed during development and found only in very low concentrations in normal adult tissues are called _____ .

4. Activated _____ destroy tumor cells *in vitro*, but do not destroy normal healthy cells.

5. The activation of both CD4+ T cells and CD8+ T cells requires the presence of _____ molecules.

Multiple Choice: Choose the best answer.

1. Molecular biology techniques have been used to construct these to help identify tumor antigens.

    a. expression libraries
    b. tumor specific antigens
    c. tumor associated antigens
    d. point mutations
    e. alterations on the cell surface

2. The sum of all products expressed by this constitutes an expression library for that malignant cell.

    a. mRNA
    b. rRNA
    c. viral DNA
    d. cDNA
    e. modified viral RNA

3. This protein has been shown to be present on cells in about half of the Hodgkin's patients.

    a. galactin 9
    b. 17-1A
    c. MAGE 1-3
    d. receptor idiotype
    e. gp120

4. All of the following are clinically important tumor associated oncofetal antigens except

    a. alpha-fetoprotein (AFP).
    b. beta-human chorionic gonadotrophin (B-HCG).
    c. Type 1 cytokines.
    d. carcinoembryonic antigen (CEA).
    e. all of the above except for b.

CRITICAL THINKING/CASE STUDY EXERCISE

The nursing class is covering hemopoiesis and the myeloid and lymphoid stem cells giving rise to formed elements of the blood, while the immunology class just finished Chapter 26 on tumor immunology. At lunch an active discussion ensues between the classes as they figure out they share a lot of similar information on certain pathologies.

1. What "certain pathologies" might the classes have talked about? How would one organize these malignancies of blood cells?

2. How would immunophenotyping analysis be used? What is the Philadelphia chromosome?

3. Distinguish myeloid and lymphoid neoplasms by describing acute and chronic leukemias, lymphocytic and myelogenous leukemias, lymphomas, and multiple myelomas. How do tumors escape the immune system?

CHAPTER 27

IMMUNODEFICIENCY DISORDERS

OUTLINE

OBJECTIVES

Upon completion of this chapter, the reader should be able to:

1. Explain the differences between primary immunodeficiency disorders and secondary immunodeficiency disorders.

2. Describe the basic genetic defect and clinical manifestations of various primary immunodeficiency disorders arising from defects in B cell development or activation.

3. Describe the basic genetic defect and clinical manifestations of primary immunodeficiency disorders arising from defects in T cell development.

4. Describe the basic genetic defect and clinical manifestations of various primary immunodeficiency disorders arising from defects in both the B cell and T cell lineages, and their function.

5. Describe the basic genetic defect and clinical manifestations of various primary immunodeficiency disorders arising from defects in biochemical processes in phagocytes.

6. Describe the basic genetic defect and clinical manifestations of various primary immunodeficiency disorders arising from defects in various complement proteins.

7. Describe the various mechanisms by which secondary immunodeficiency disorders arise.

SUMMARY OF KEY POINTS

Immunodeficiency disorders result in decreased host resistance to some types of infection, and they are classed as either primary or secondary. Primary immunodeficiency disorders are inherited, and secondary immunodeficiency disorders are acquired.

The most common immunodeficiency disorders are inherited B cell disorders. *X-linked agammaglobulinemia* (XLA) or *Bruton's agammaglobulinemia* is an immunodeficiency B cell disorder linked to the X chromosome, which results from a single gene encoding a tyrosine kinase important for signaling. Without the signaling, the preB cells do not develop to mature B cells. A gross deficiency or absence of mature B cells occurs. *Selective IgA deficiency* is the most common of the immunodeficiency disorders in which increased incidence of recurrent sinopulmonary infection, increased association with allergies, and gastrointestinal disease are observed. About half of the individuals with this defect are asymptomatic, however. *Immunoglobulin deficiency with increased IgM* is a primary immunodeficiency disorder in which there is an increased serum level of IgM but a decrease in IgG, IgA, and IgE due to the decreased expression of CD40L on T cells whose interaction is required for B cell activation.

Primary immunodeficiency T cell disorders are rare, but the prototypic inherited T cell disorder is *DiGeorge's syndrome* or thymic hypoplasia, which results from defective embryogenesis leading to a reduced and defective (or absent) thymus. Therapy for DiGeorge's syndrome is fetal thymic tissue fragment transplantation placed under the renal capsule. Individuals improve with age due to development presumably from extrathymic maturation sites.

Combined T cell and B cell disorders manifest when there are deficits in the bone marrow progenitor cells that give rise to both T cells and B cells. The prototypic immunodeficiency disorder affecting both T cells and B cells is *severe combined immunodeficiency* (SCID). SCID can result from different etiologies, but a defect in the enzyme, adenosine deaminase (ADA), occurs in about 50% of the cases. The genetic defect is not known for many SCID cases. *Wiskott Aldrich syndrome* (WAS) is an X-linked primary immunodeficiency involving both T cells and B cells in which the genetic defect is encoded on the X chromosome. The protein has been named the Wiskott Aldrich syndrome protein (WASP), and point mutation in the gene has been isolated in patients with WAS. WASP interacts with a protein involved in cytoskeletal reorganization.

Phagocytic disorders represent approximately 20% of immunodeficiency disorders. *Chronic granulomatous disease* (CGD) is a phagocytic disorder resulting from a genetic defect in the NADPH oxidase complex that is required for the production of reactive oxygen intermediates within the phagocytic vacuole. These reactive oxygen intermediates are cytotoxic to microbes inside the phagocytic vacuole. *Chediak Higashi syndrome* is a multi-system immunodeficiency disorder in which patients are susceptible to a variety of pathogens including bacteria, fungi, and viruses. This susceptibility is primarily the result of dysfunctional neutrophils. Chediak Higashi syndrome is recognized by the presence of giant cytoplasmic granules occurring as a result of uncontrolled granule membrane fusion. Natural killer cell function is decreased in these patients, probably because of the inability of the natural killer cells to release granules containing perforin. *Leukocyte adhesion deficiency* (LAD) is a disorder in which leukocytes lack or have a low-level expression of CD18 molecules, which make up the beta chain of a class of heterodimeric adhesion molecules. Neutrophils are especially affected because they do not express compensatory adhesive molecules to allow migration into tissues at sites of inflammation. An elevated blood neutrophil count is a consequence, as well as an inability to form pus efficiently, and poor wound healing. When expression is totally absent, patients may die within the first year of life, but low-level expression is more common.

Bacterial infections and autoimmunity are frequently associated with complement system defects, and defects in almost all components of the complement system and regulatory proteins have been described. The most serious complement defect is of the complement protein C3. Patients with a deficiency in the C1 inhibitor protein often present with life-threatening edema called *hereditary angioneurotic edema*, while deficiencies of C1, C2, or C4 do not usually present a clinical problem when the alternative pathway of complement is intact. Deficiencies of the C5-C0 complement proteins lead to increased susceptibility to *Neisseria spp.* infections. *Decay accelerating factor* (DAF) and *CD59* are regulatory complement proteins linked to red blood cells via GPI linkages. In *paroxysmal nocturnal hemoglobinuria*, red blood cells do not express DAF or CD59 because they are unable to make the GPI linkages, and as a result they are susceptible to lysis by complement.

Causes of secondary immunodeficiency disorders are diverse, ranging from acquired immunodeficiency diseases to chosen lifestyles and normal physiological changes. Viral infections (e.g., HIV), therapeutic drugs, malnutrition and diseases, normal physiological changes, and abnormal production of immunological effectors all result in acquired immunodeficiency disorders.

REVIEW OF KEY TERMS AND ABBREVIATIONS

Matching: Match the key term in the left column with the definition in the right column.

1. _____ adenosine deaminase

2. _____ B cell disorders

3. _____ Bruton's

4. _____ C1 inhibitor

5. _____ CD55

6. _____ Chediak Higashi

7. _____ DAF

a) also known as CD55

b) membrane attack complexes on red blood cells

c) life-threatening edema

d) X-linked; involves T and B cells

e) inherited disorders

f) enzyme replacement for ADA-SCID

g) essential substances lacking in one's diet

8. _____ DiGeorge's

9. _____ HANE

10. _____ LAD

11. _____ malnutrition

12. _____ PNH

13. _____ primary

14. _____ secondary

15. _____ SCID

16. _____ WAS

17. _____ WASP

18. _____ therapeutic gamma globulin

19. _____ PEG-ADA

h) acquired disorders result of disease, etc.

i) regulatory complement protein

j) protein encoded on X chromosome

k) X-linked agammaglobulinemia

l) injection of gamma globulin from donor serum

m) defects in this enzyme can lead to SCID

n) affects both T cells and B cells

o) associated with T cell immunity

p) regulatory protein

q) phagocytes lack cell surface molecules

r) giant cytoplasmic granules associated with this

s) most common primary immunodeficiency

Definitions: Write the definition of each of the following words or terms.

1. Bruton's agammaglobulinemia _____

_____

2. CD55 _____

_____

3. Chediak Higashi syndrome _____

_____

4. DiGeorge's syndrome _____

_____

5. giant cytoplasmic granules _____

_____

6. hereditary angioneurotic edema _____

_____

7. immunoglobulin deficiency with increased IgM _____

_____

8. leukocyte adhesion deficiency _____

_____

9. malnutrition _____

_____

10. paroxysmal nocturnal hemoglobinuria _____

_____

11. severe combined immunodeficiency disorders _____

_____

12. therapeutic gamma globulin _____

_____

13. selective IgA deficiency _____

_____

REVIEW EXERCISES

True or False: Read each statement and decide if it is TRUE or FALSE. Place T or F on the line before each statement.

1. _____   Immunodeficiency disorders are classified as primary or secondary.

2. _____   Secondary disorders are inherited, while primary disorders are acquired.

3. _____   Inherited T cell disorders are the most common of their type.

4. _____   Bruton's agammaglobulinemia is a disorder linked to the Y chromosome.

5. _____   XLA results from a defect in a gene encoding a tyrosine kinase signal.

Fill in the Blank: Complete the following sentences on the immune system by filling in the missing word or words.

1. Individuals with selective IgA deficiency show an increased incidence of _____ .

2. _____ is the prototypic inherited T cell disorder.

3. Congenital thymic hypoplasia presents with a reduced, defective, absent _____ .

4. About 50% of all SCID cases are due to defects in the enzyme _____ .

5. _____ is an X-linked primary immunodeficiency involving both T and B cells.

Multiple Choice: Choose the best answer.

1. Protein encoded on X chromosome in WAS.

   a. WASP
   b. interferon gamma
   c. NADPH oxidase
   d. gp91 phox
   e. p47 phox

2. Chediak Higashi syndrome is recognized by the presence of

   a. giant cytoplasmic granules.
   b. nitroblue tetrazolium.
   c. CD34+ precursor cells.
   d. NADPH oxidase.
   e. Wiskott Aldrich syndrome protein.

3. Capsular antigens are typically

   a. B-dependent antigens.
   b. T-dependent antigens.
   c. B-independent antigens.
   d. T-independent antigens.
   e. none of the above.

4. Phagocytic disorders represent approximately _____ of immunodeficiency disorders.

   a. 40%
   b. 10%
   c. 20%
   d. less than 1%
   e. more than 50%

CRITICAL THINKING EXERCISE

Tom and Sarah are studying for a quiz tomorrow on immunodeficiency disorders, and they are fascinated by the inherited ones, especially Bruton's agammaglobulinemia. They have read about this mostly male disorder and its strange appearance at about nine months of age.

1. What is Bruton's agammaglobulinemia? Is it one of the more common immunodeficiencies?

2. Why does this genetic defect become apparent at approximately 6–9 months of age? Why are recurrent upper respiratory infections the manifestation? What is the treatment?

3. What would a measurement of serum immunoglobulin reveal in Bruton's agammaglobulinemia?

HYPERSENSITIVITY

OUTLINE

OBJECTIVES

Upon completion of this chapter, the reader should be able to:

1. List the Gell and Coombs classification scheme for hypersensitivity reactions.
2. Briefly describe the general characteristics, sensitization phase, effector phase, and clinical manifestations of Type I hypersensitivity reactions.
3. Briefly describe the general characteristics, sensitization phase, effector phase, and clinical manifestations of Type II hypersensitivity reactions.
4. Briefly describe the general characteristics, sensitization phase, effector phase, and clinical manifestations of Type III hypersensitivity reactions.
5. Briefly describe the general characteristics, sensitization phase, effector phase, and clinical manifestations of Type IV hypersensitivity reactions.
6. Describe RAST laboratory test and its limitations as a diagnostic tool for allergen specific IgE.

SUMMARY OF KEY POINTS

Normal immunological responses not controlled by regulatory mechanisms are hypersensitivity reactions, and are generally classed using the Gell and Coombs system, or modified version of it, and include Type I-immediate hypersensitivity, Type II-antibody mediated, Type III-immune complex mediated, and Type IV-T cell mediated.

Type I hypersensitivity reactions are also called immediate hypersensitivity or IgE-mediated reactions, and they manifest clinically as allergies, rhinitis, or anaphylaxis. Two distinct phases are seen in the development of immediate hypersensitivity: sensitization and effector phases. The sensitization phase is the immunological phase marked by the production of antigen specific IgE antibodies that bond to mast cells or basophils by their Fc regions. The effector phase is the pathological phase marked by inflammation following degranulation of mast cells and basophils when the Fab regions are crosslinked by antigen. Localized reactions include allergic rhinitis and asthma, and anaphylaxis is a systemic and potentially fatal immediate hypersensitivity response. Effectiveness of allergy shots or desensitization therapy is controversial. The RAST test determines the presence of serum IgE antibodies specific for an antigen, but the limitation of this test is that most of the IgE is bound to the mast cells and basophils and not in the serum. IgE bound to mast cells and basophils is therefore not detected.

Type II hypersensitivity reactions are antibody mediated, and in contrast to immediate hypersensitivity reactions, antibodies participating in Type II hypersensitivity responses are IgG and IgM antibodies. These antibodies bind to antigens on cell surfaces. The effector phase includes complement activation, natural killer cell antibody dependent cell mediated cytotoxicity (ADCC), and opsonin mediated phagocytosis. All these processes destroy the cell expressing their target antigen. Type II hypersensitivity reactions can lead to a wide spectrum of clinical manifestations depending on the cell type expressing the antigen, and include hemolytic disease of the newborn, autoimmune disorders, drug-induced reactions, and transfusion reactions.

Type III hypersensitivity reactions are also mediated following the generation of IgG and IgM antibodies, but Type III reactions differ from Type II reactions in that the antigen is soluble and soluble immune complexes are formed. The effector phase of Type II hypersensitivity reactions becomes apparent when the number of immune complexes formed overwhelms the clearance mechanisms. As number and size of immune complexes increase, they deposit in capillary walls and are immobilized there. Immune complexes play a primary pathologic role in some systemic diseases according to an overwhelming body of evidence including systemic lupus erythematosus (SLE), post streptococcal glomerulonephritis, serum sickness, and farmer's lung.

Type IV hypersensitivity responses are cell mediated, and antibodies do not play a part in these responses. The effector phase of Type IV hypersensitivity reactions are also called delayed type hypersensitivity (DTH) responses. The sensitization phase of Type IV hypersensitivity reactions is initiated when naïve CD4+ T cells are activated in response to a class II MHC-antigenic peptide on the surface of an antigen presenting cell. The effector phase is initiated when memory CD4+ T cells are activated during their immunosurveillance. Type I cytokines (e.g., IFNγ and TNF) secreted by activated CD4+ T cells enhance the cytotoxicity of macrophages leading to more inflammatory mediator release and observed DTH response. DTH response can be chronic (chronic infection with *Mycobacterium tuberculosis*) or acute (prototypic acute DTH response is the Mantoux test referred to as the tuberculosis test). Contact sensitivity is a variant DTH response, so poison ivy dermatitis is the prototypic contact sensitivity response. Contact sensitivity reactions can also occur in response to various metals in jewelry.

REVIEW OF KEY TERMS AND ABBREVIATIONS

Matching: Match the key term in the left column with the definition in the right column.

1. _____ hypersensitivity

2. _____ Type I

3. _____ anaphylaxis

4. _____ desensitization

5. _____ C5a

6. _____ C3b

7. _____ Type II

8. _____ haptens

9. _____ IgM antibodies

10. _____ Type III

11. _____ Type IV

12. _____ serum sickness

13. _____ DTH

a) HDN, autoimmune disorders, drug and transfusion reactions

b) chemoattractant for neutrophils

c) determines allergen specific IgE in serum

d) cytotoxic to *M. tuberculosis* in phagocytic vacuole

e) allergies, rhinitis, anaphylaxis

f) responses not controlled by normal regulatory mechanisms

g) IgG and IgM target soluble antigens; complexes form

h) effector phase of Type IV reactions

i) contact sensitivity or dermatitis; variant DTH response

j) too small to trigger an immune response

k) allergen extracts are separated by gel electrophoresis

l) T cell mediated

m) potentially fatal immediate hypersensitivity, cardiac, respiratory

14. _____ Mantoux test

    n) facilitates phagocytosis by functioning as an opsonin

15. _____ nitric oxide

    o) isohemagglutinins

16. _____ poison ivy

    p) non human gamma globulin for passive immunization

17. _____ RAST

    q) allergy shots; antigen in small doses triggers isotype switching

18. _____ immunoblot

    r) is a DTH skin test for *Mycobacterium tuberculosis* exposure

Definitions: Write the definition of each of the following words or terms.

1. hypersensitivity reactions _____

_____

2. Type I _____

_____

3. Type II _____

_____

4. Type III _____

_____

5. Type IV _____

_____

6. anaphylaxis _____

_____

7. desensitization _____

_____

8. hemolytic disease of the newborn _____

_____

9. haptens _____

_____

10. Goodpasture's syndrome _____

_____

11. myasthenia gravis _____

_____

12. isohemagglutinins _____

_____

REVIEW EXERCISES

True or False: Read each statement and decide if it is TRUE or FALSE. Place T or F on the line before each statement.

1. _____ Hypersensitivity reactions are immunological responses controlled by normal regulatory mechanisms.

2. _____ Allergic reactions are the most common manifestation of Type I hypersensitivity reactions.

3. _____ Atopy is a term used to refer to IgA mediated allergic reactions.

4. _____ Initial immunological response following exposure to an antigen constitutes the desensitization phase.

5. _____ Most of the IgE formed binds to FcεR present on mast cells and basophils normally.

Fill in the Blank: Complete the following sentences on the immune system by filling in the missing word or words.

1. _____ are the circulating mast cell counterpart.

2. _____ are found around blood vessels in connective tissue.

3. _____ is a potentially fatal immediate hypersensitivity response with both cardiac and respiratory symptoms.

4. Individuals at risk for anaphylaxis should carry _____ .

5. _____ acts on the vascular endothelium causing an increase in vascular permeability.

Multiple Choice: Choose the best answer.

1. A pharmacological agent that stabilizes the mast cell/basophil membrane is

    a. epinephrine.
    b. allergy shots.
    c. histamine.
    d. anti-histamine.
    e. sodium cromoglycate.

2. Desensitization treatments are commonly referred to as

    a. isotype switching.
    b. allergy shots.
    c. epi-pen.
    d. histamine.
    e. anti-histamine.

3. Chemoattractant for neutrophils is

    a. chemotaxis.
    b. C3b.
    c. C5a.
    d. histamine.
    e. epinephrine.

4. Hemolytic disease of the newborn occurs when a mother, whose red blood cells do not express the Rh antigen, is carrying a fetus that is

    a. Rh negative.
    b. Rh neutral.
    c. Rh positive.
    d. anti-Rh.
    e. none of the above.

CRITICAL THINKING EXERCISE

The immunology class is elated at finishing the class, but is having a difficult time figuring out the different types of hypersensitivity reactions. Most of the class knows about allergies, anaphylaxis, and things like contact dermatitis firsthand, but some of the other hypersensitivity reactions are somewhat vague to them.

1. How would the Gell and Coombs system help the students understand hypersensitivity reactions?

2. Where would the things they do understand fit in the Gell and Coombs system? What are sensitization and effector phases, and how might they help the students?

3. What are atopic individuals and what is one of the contributing factors in the switch to IgE? What are prophylactic treatments for atopic individuals? What type of hypersensitivity reaction do transplants represent? persistent infections? delayed type hypersensitivity (DTH) response?

ANSWER KEY

CHAPTER 1

Matching

1. k
2. t
3. g
4. o
5. q
6. c
7. m
8. a
9. n
10. h
11. p
12. e
13. j
14. b
15. f
16. l
17. r
18. u
19. i
20. d
21. s

Definitions

1. Membrane antibodies are antibodies expressed on the outside of antigen presenting cells like B cells.
2. Membrane immunoglobulins are membrane antibodies; synonymous term.
3. Mucous membranes refer to the epithelial coverings that line all anatomical openings to the outside world.
4. Natural killer cells are part of the innate immunity of the body, and are cellular components not specific to a particular antigen. Compare with cytotoxic killer cells.
5. Mast cells develop from basophils, which leave the capillaries and enter other tissue. Mast cells liberate histamine, serotonin, and heparin.
6. Pepsin is a chemical substance of innate immunity acting in the stomach's acidic environment. It is a proteolytic (protein-digesting) gastric enzyme.
7. Phagocytes include neutrophils, monocytes, and macrophages that ingest microbes and foreign debris they may encounter in the body. Part of innate immunity.
8. Plasma cells proliferate from B cells. While B cells exhibit antibodies on their plasma membranes, the plasma cells, which are derived from the B cells, actually secrete the antibodies.

9. Recognition is the immune system's ability to tell self from non-self. It is one of the two main characteristics of immunity; the other being "getting rid of non-self".
10. Resident flora refers to the normal bacteria and fungi inhabiting in and on the body.
11. Skin refers to the cutaneous membrane that maintains the body's physical and biochemical integrity. The skin is part of the innate immunity.
12. Stomach acidity is part of innate immunity, killing many potential pathogens.
13. T cells develop in bone marrow and mature in the thymus to become important cellular components of adaptive immunity.

True or False

1. False
2. False
3. True
4. False
5. True

Fill in the Blank

1. recognition
2. resident flora
3. plasma cells
4. cytotoxic killer T cells
5. Helper T cells

Multiple Choice

1. d
2. e
3. a
4. b
5. c

Critical Thinking 1

1. You would point out to Tom that adaptive immunity "adapts" to whatever antigen it encounters. Tom probably got the term "acquired" from earlier interpretations.
2. Explain to Tom that immunity is one complex process involving lots of different chemical substances, cells, and tissues, but those innate and adaptive processes are only separated to make it easier to teach. It is academic, not two processes.
3. Most of the research into immunity has focused on adaptive immunity, so the emphasis historically has been on specificity. Several things may change Tom's mind about thinking this way. Cytokines are probably one of the easiest ways to see the interrelatedness of the two academic divisions of immunity.

Critical Thinking 2

1. The class of helper T cell and the individual type of cytokine will determine the outcome or resolution of an infection. Without recognition, a resolution is impossible; but resolution shapes the future of any potential for recognition.
2. All this incredible variation allows for an almost infinite set of immune responses in the form of antibodies specific to whatever antigen is presented. In order to recognize an antigen, a particular antibody with its receptor has to be present.
3. Without antigen presenting cells no recognition would ever occur!

Critical Thinking 3

1. Tom and Sarah are not seeing the "big picture." They missed out on the preliminary discussion in the chapter on the academic and arbitrary separation of immunity into two processes or divisions.
2. The complexity may seem overwhelming, but the lists of chemical substances, cellular factors, and tissues are simply in the text to help you analyze how immunity works. Seeing the whole working together and interacting, not one part or process independent of any other parts or processes, embraces innate and adaptive immunity.
3. Tom wants to place all the processes into two categories only. He encounters a big problem with that when "humoral" and "cellular components" come up. Tom would like to place both these into one or the other of the two arbitrary processes, but he cannot do it. If you see both innate and adaptive processes working together, it is much easier to see humoral and cellular components as being shared elements in immune system functions.

Case Study

1. Saying it was "just a virus" tells us precious little about what sort of pathogen it may be or what antigen(s) it may possess.
2. Tissues involved would certainly include the mucous membranes of the respiratory and digestive tracts, although the headache, fever, and general body aches hint at nervous system involvement as well. Cells of both innate as well as adaptive immunity are involved like phagocytes and lymphocytes respectively. Lysozymes, mucus, and gastric secretions from innate immunity, as well as cytokines from adaptive immunity are definitely involved.
3. Descriptions would include mucus production and cilia movement for innate immunity, and T and B lymphocyte production as the illness progresses over several days. While it is impossible to accurately predict whether the clinician will succumb to this same identical "virus" again, you can make several observations. One observation is that since the clinician reports these signs and symptoms every other year or so, either the "virus" changes its antigenic character and thus avoids any adaptive memory mechanism, or another, but very similar, "virus" is introduced every other year or so for which the adaptive immune system of the clinician is unprepared. The assumption throughout is that the clinician's immune system is not suppressed and (s)he is healthy, and we are not considering lifestyle or chemical problems with immunity. Stress or emotional factors could be part of this pattern of recurring illness, too, especially if there is a temporal or seasonal correlation of the illness with work or personal life events. Distress could suppress an otherwise healthy immune system making the clinician an easy target "every year or so."

CHAPTER 2

Matching

1. g
2. o
3. a
4. k
5. n
6. e
7. r
8. s
9. m

10. f
11. t
12. i
13. q
14. l
15. h
16. c
17. u
18. j
19. b
20. d
21. p

Definitions

1. A tumor specific antigen is a protein different from all others in the genetic code.
2. T-dependent antigens require T cells to be present to activate B cells.
3. T-independent antigens activate B cells in the absence of T cells.
4. Con A refers to concanavalin A, which is a plant glycoprotein that activates T cells (polyclonal activator).
5. LPS refers to lipopolysaccharide, which polyclonally activates B cells.
6. MHC refers to the major histocompatibility complex. Unique proteins are encoded by this gene complex. T cells recognize epitopes on antigen fragments bound to these unique proteins. These proteins act as potent antigens when introduced into another individual.
7. PHA refers to polyhemagglutinin, which is a plant glycoprotein that activates T cells (polyclonal activator).
8. PWM refers to pokeweed mitogen, which polyclonally activates both T cells and B cells.
9. Haptens are small molecules which are not of themselves immunogenic, but when coupled to a high molecular weight substance can become immunogenic. In effect, a hapten becomes an epitope associated with the carrier to form a hapten-carrier complex.
10. Epitopes are specific regions of an antigen referred to as antigenic determinants that are the only regions recognized by the antigen receptors of B cells and T cells.
11. Adjuvants are enhancers of immunogenicity for vaccines. These substances improve the immune response to an antigen by keeping the antigen in the system longer through surrounding it. That way, the antigen remains for a longer period of time stimulating appropriate immune cells including phagocytes. Examples of adjuvants include alum precipitate, MF-59 with squaline, and Freund's complete adjuvant with killed *Mycobacterium tuberculosis*.
12. A carrier is a high molecular weight protein, which by attaching to a smaller molecule called a hapten, allows the hapten to become immunogenic, becoming a hapten-carrier complex.
13. Opsonin is a generic term for molecules that bind antigens for indirect mode recognition. Opsonins serve as a link between an innate immunity cell and an antigen.

True or False

1. True
2. True
3. False
4. True
5. False

Fill in the Blank

1. antigens
2. Superantigens/oligoclonal activators
3. opsonin
4. intact
5. specificity

Multiple Choice

1. c
2. a
3. c
4. d
5. d

Critical Thinking 1

1. Tom and Sarah explain that polysaccharides can be immunogenic under certain circumstances like being large, foreign, and attached to a protein complex, and that in this chapter they have just learned that the polysaccharides present on red blood cells are immunogenic.

   The obvious problem to Tom and Sarah (if not seen yet by the nursing students) is that the antigens on red blood cells will form complexes with antibodies present in other types of blood in the ABO system. This will be a major problem if the wrong blood types are mixed in a transfusion and they clump up (agglutinate) in blood vessels.
2. Polysaccharides are not the most immunogenic of molecules; proteins are the most immunogenic, however, because they are complex, large, and foreign. It is a unique and somewhat mysterious characteristic of red blood cells (erythrocytes) that polysaccharides attached to the cell membrane are immunogenic.
3. Probably to put all this together Tom and Sarah will have to understand what these biological polymers are in the first place: polysaccharides, proteins, lipids, and nucleic acids. (In order to understand proteins are complex, Sarah, Tom, and the nursing students will have to understand at least that there are twenty different building blocks/monomers/amino acids to choose from in different orders and sequences and levels of complexity making proteins most immunogenic of the biological polymers; while polysaccharides will be seen to be large and they certainly can be foreign, but the units that repeat are amazingly similar, and not complex at all.)

Critical Thinking 2

1. Sarah may challenge Tom to tell her about direct versus indirect recognition for innate immunity, and to elaborate (if he is able to) on how different the receptors of direct recognition by innate immune cells are from that of adaptive immune cells. That would really demonstrate if Tom could realize differences and similarities between innate and adaptive immunity.
2. Opsonins are unique to the indirect recognition of innate immune cells, especially phagocytes, natural killer cells, mast cells, and basophils. Another molecule (opsonin) binds the antigen and drags it along to the innate immune cell that recognizes the opsonin (serving as the link to the antigen). Adaptive immune cells (B cells and T cells) recognize the antigen without benefit of the opsonin, yet in different ways: B cells recognize epitopes on intact antigens, while T cells recognize epitopes on antigen fragments bound to unique proteins. B cells and T cells recognize epitopes since they only interact with that part when binding antigen.

3. The proteins that bind the antigen fragments and their epitopes recognized by T cells are encoded by a special gene complex referred to as the major histocompatibility complex (MHC). These proteins are potent antigens in their own right when introduced into another individual. After antigens are degraded enzymatically into small peptide pieces by antigen presenting cells, these peptides are bound to the MHC proteins where they are displayed for T cells to recognize along with the protein as a whole. There are two types of MHC proteins, one type for cytotoxic T cells and the second type recognized by helper T cells.

Case Study

1. Sarah and Tom have learned that antigens are monoclonal activators that stimulate cells expressing antigen receptors specific for an epitope. T cells or B cells that are activated after contact with an antigen proliferate into a population of cells forming one (mono) clone. The connection to a class of antibodies created specifically from plasma cells coming from differentiated B cells is obvious. Each of these unique antibodies forms unique receptors for each unique antigen epitope, and binds it. Tom and Sarah see that monoclonal antibodies could easily be used to check for binding (agglutination) of specific antigens (e.g., hepatitis viruses and strep throat). Sarah and Tom also realize that in special physiological scenarios someone may express a particular protein (like a hormone or enzyme) that could be checked with a monoclonal antibody specific to it; pregnancy tests work like this in which the hormone, human chorionic gonadotropin, is checked for by antibodies, which will complex with it and produce a color change.
2. In disease states like autoimmunity, the immune system responds to body proteins as if they were foreign. Body proteins may not be foreign, and yet be immunogenic. Furthermore, cancer cells with genetic mutations do express proteins that are seen as foreign by the immune system even though produced by previously normal body cells. Tom and Sarah know that when these mutations result in proteins expressed different from all other ones expressed by the genetic code, then that protein is called tumor specific antigen. The same sort of interaction that one would see with monoclonal antibodies for specific antigens would be possible for detection of tumor specific antigens, and the spread of cancer (metastasis) could possibly be monitored in this manner, too. Knowing how much and how fast a cancer was spreading would be useful in treatment options and in making an informed prognosis.
3. Sarah and Tom can tell the technician that polyclonal activators are typically plant proteins binding to virtually all T cells and/or B cells. Many (poly) clones are generated by this binding. Plant glycoproteins activating T cells are polyhemagglutinin (PHA) and concanavalin A (Con A), while pokeweed mitogen (PWM) activates both T cells and B cells.

   The lab is probably very interested in any source of antibodies, especially polyclonal activators because there is a larger source of potential antibodies to begin with and a greater likelihood of eliciting some sort of a response from a B cell activation. Of course, the diversity of populations of cells could also present a bewildering array of possibilities as well. With careful isolation and characterization, however, the polyclonal activators or mitogens present many opportunities in research: a sort of "job security!"

CHAPTER 3

Matching

1. i
2. m
3. a

4. o
5. f
6. k
7. c
8. e
9. j
10. b
11. g
12. d
13. p
14. n
15. h
16. l
17. s
18. q
19. u
20. r
21. t

Definitions

1. Bifunctional refers to the fact that antibodies have both an antigen-binding domain and a separate domain that determines other biological activities.
2. Electrophoresis is the separation of proteins while under the influence of an electric field. Five distinct bands can be detected in this manner with blood serum proteins.
3. A hybridoma is a biological "factory" for production of an antibody of a given specificity and isotype. A hybrid cell is created from the fusion of two cells, one a normal spleen-derived plasma cell, and the other commercially available malignant plasma cell that does not secrete antibodies. The immortality of the myeloma and the specificity and isotype of the normal plasma cell component combine to form the "factory."
4. Isotype refers to the antibody (immunoglobulin) heavy chain constant regions (IgM, IgD, IgG, IgE, and IgA).
5. Monoclonal refers to antibodies specific for one epitope.
6. The variable region of an antibody is the component of the antibody that provides its specificity.
7. The constant region is the component of an antibody that does not vary.
8. Affinity is the association constant between antibody and a univalent antigen.
9. Avidity is a measure of the overall binding between the antigen-binding sites and multivalent antigen.
10. An antibody is an immunoglobulin or protein playing a major role in immune responses. They may be on the surface of B cells or a differentiated form of a B cell, plasma cells may secrete them.
11. Cross-reactivity refers to the phenomenon in which some antibodies secreted by one plasma cell can bind to a similar, but not identical epitope.
12. Differentiation refers to the phenomenon in which B cells are activated by an antigen to become transformed into plasma cells secreting antibodies specific to the activating antigen.
13. Major basic protein is a protein released by eosinophils that is cytotoxic to helminths.

True or False

1. False
2. True
3. False

4. True
5. True

Fill in the Blank

1. antigen
2. affinity
3. zeta
4. isotypes
5. opsonins

Multiple Choice

1. e
2. b
3. e
4. a
5. a

Critical Thinking 1

1. Infection with the bacteria, *Clostridium tetani*, leads to a systemic tetanic contraction (lockjaw) that is often fatal. A protein, tetanus toxin, is secreted by *Clostridium tetani*, which causes the spasmodic contractions.
2. Toxoid is a laboratory-modified form of the toxin. Toxoid is used in lieu of the toxin because the toxin dose required to get an immune response is in excess of lethality.
3. The anti-toxoid antibodies are cross-reactive with the toxin, and these anti-toxoid antibodies will bind to, and neutralize the toxin. Therefore, exposure to toxins will not cause lockjaw because the anti-toxoid antibodies will bind to, and neutralize the toxin.

Critical Thinking 2

1. Kim and Sarah also need to know that the classic monomeric antibody has two identical heavy chains connected to each other by disulfide bridges, and with variable regions where antigen binding takes place (2 segments on light chains and 3 segments on heavy chains). Specificity is conferred upon this classic monomeric antibody by the two identical binding sites it has. Antibodies also have five potential constant regions in separate domains that determine other biological activities.
2. B cells are activated by an antigen which causes their transformation and differentiation into antibody-secreting plasma cells specific to the activating antigen.
3. Neutralization of viruses is one example of material Tom neglected to mention. (There are others like biological activities mentioned in more detail below.) In neutralization, antibodies bind to the domain of viruses that ordinarily allows them to bind and enter into potential host cells, and this is an important aspect of this antibody/antigen binding Tom failed to mention.

Critical Thinking 3

1. Avidity is the measure of overall binding between the antigen-binding sites and multivalent antigen, whereas affinity is the association constant between antibody and a univalent antigen. Different sets of antibodies bind to the same epitope with different binding strengths or avidities. One antibody will have a better "goodness of fit."
2. Pepsin and papain, proteolytic enzymes from gastric juice and papaya, digest the polypeptide chains in antibodies into fragments. Papain treatment yields three fragments (two termed **Fab** = fragment

antigen binding, and **Fc** = fragment crystallizable), and treatment with pepsin yields only one major fragment (two Fab sites in a single structure and the Fc degraded). The Fab fragment binds antigen, and the Fc is required for the biological functions of antibodies.

3. The antibody fragments play a role in bifunctionality (biological functions domain versus antigen-binding site domain). Some examples of biological functions include binding of Fc receptors and complement fixation.

Case Study

1. Was Aunt Margaret's first pregnancy with a Rh+ child? Does she know the Rh factor yet of her second pregnancy? Sarah, knowing about the antibody problems of Rh– mothers with Rh+ children, would want to know the answers to the previous questions. No potential problems would exist until the second such pregnancy, since maternal blood can only encounter the newborn's blood at birth when such a mixing could occur in the first pregnancy. Antibodies produced then by the mother are circulating and ready to cross the placenta in subsequent pregnancies.

2. Benefits of antibodies and pregnancy include IgG antibodies crossing the placenta crucial for fetal immunity.

3. Precautionary RhoGAM administered by the clinician as soon as it is recognized that a Rh– mother is carrying a Rh+ child precludes any problems such as HDN (hemolytic disease of the newborn), since it prevents the antibody formation (anti-Rh antibody) that could harm another Rh+ child in subsequent pregnancies.

CHAPTER 4

Matching

1. h
2. u
3. a
4. n
5. q
6. s
7. t
8. j
9. p
10. k
11. g
12. c
13. l
14. r
15. i
16. m
17. b
18. f
19. d
20. o
21. e

Definitions

1. Bursa of Fabricius refers to the site in birds in which B cell maturation was discovered first.
2. Cutaneous immune system refers to immune cells located just below the skin.
3. Eosinophil cationic protein is a toxic protein.
4. Interferon gamma is a cytokine enhancing the cytotoxic ability of the activated macrophage.
5. Keratinocytes are cells in the epidermis producing a number of molecules playing a role in host defense.
6. Killer inhibitory receptor (KIR) refers to recognition of some type I major histocompatibility complex proteins on the surface of cells.
7. Langerhan's cells are antigen-presenting cells in the epidermis.
8. Lymph nodes are small encapsulated structures located at the junction of the main lymphatic tracts.
9. Lymphoid refers to the lineage of self-renewing precursor cells giving rise to mature B cells and pre-T cells.
10. Myeloid refers to the lineage of self-renewing precursor cells giving rise to neutrophils, monocytes, basophils, and eosinophils.
11. Mast cells are cells in connective tissue, gastrointestinal tract, blood vessels, and mucosal epithelium responsible for inflammatory response.
12. Peyer's patches refers to a region in the gut where lymphoid follicles are aggregated.
13. Phagolysosome refers to a chimeric vacuole resulting from fusion of cytosolic lysosomes with the phagosome.

True or False

1. True
2. False
3. True
4. True
5. False

Fill in the Blank

1. phagolysosome
2. primitive pattern recognition receptors
3. respiratory burst
4. thymic selection
5. perforin

Multiple Choice

1. c
2. d
3. a
4. c
5. a

Critical Thinking 1

1. Dendritic cells are cells with the ability to engulf antigens, degrade them, and display antigen fragments on the cell surface in association with major histocompatibility complex proteins; also known as antigen-presenting cells. Tom is referring to cells in the epidermis with long projections (Langerhan's cells) with which they .pick up antigens coming through the skin.

2. Dendritic cell and antigen-presenting cell are synonymous, and Langerhan's cells and other antigen-presenting cells (macrophages and B cells) work together.
3. The special cells in the epidermis are referred to as Langerhan's cells, although a special class of T cells is present and helper T cells, cytotoxic T cells, and macrophages are in the dermis.

Critical Thinking 2

1. Kim is correct in saying that phagocytes can interact directly with microorganisms, but Tom is right, too, when he asserts they interact indirectly via opsonins. Phagocytes can interact directly through primitive pattern recognition receptors (PPRP) that recognize a wide array of molecules that may be present on the surface of microorganisms.
2. Phagocytes have been shown to interact indirectly with microorganisms when opsonins have been deposited on the microbial cell surface. Ingestion occurs when the macrophage extends its finger-like projections around the antigen forming a vesicle in the cytosol called a phagosome.
3. Common opsonins are the IgG antibodies, a protein (C3b), and CRP secreted by hepatocytes.

Critical Thinking 3

1. Eosinophils arise from progenitor cells (myeloid) in bone marrow. Eosinophils are included in the list of cells of innate immunity.
2. Eosinophils are the main host defense mechanism in response to parasitic infections, particularly helminths.
3. Eosinophils bind the Fc region of IgE antibodies bound to helminths, and then release major basic protein and eosinophil cationic protein that are toxic to the helminth.

Case Study

1. Chronic granulomatous disease (CGD) is a hereditary disorder whereby sufferers are unable to produce reactive oxygen intermediates (respiratory burst) due to a defective NADPH oxidase.
2. A simple, qualitative test, the nitroblue tetrazolium (NBT) slide test, can be used to assess whether NADPH oxidase is functional. NBT is a clear yellow water-soluble substance that changes to a deep dark blue/black precipitate during activation of phagocytosis. Absence of color change indicates a genetic defect in a patient in recurrent infections. The precipitate may be extracted, solubilized, and measured for a quantitative spectrophotometric test.
3. Antibiotics are prescribed for CGD, but with increase in antibiotic resistance, some infections become life-threatening. Gene therapy, in which the normal counterpart of the defective gene is introduced into the patient suffering from CGD, offers the most hope for future treatment; and already some patients have been successfully treated this way.

CHAPTER 5

Matching

1. m
2. a
3. q
4. j
5. h
6. o
7. s

8. f
9. r
10. n
11. i
12. t
13. e
14. p
15. u
16. k
17. l
18. b
19. c
20. d
21. g

Definitions

1. B cell maturation refers to the progressive expression of cell surface proteins on a cell until the cell matures to the point that it can participate in host defense.
2. B cell receptor refers to a membrane-bound antibody or membrane immunoglobulin that can recognize an antigenic epitope.
3. B cell repertoire refers to diversity of receptors or antibody diversity.
4. Lipopolysaccharide refers to the outer membrane of gram negative bacteria, which is a T-independent antigen.
5. Membrane-bound antibody refers to B cell receptors.
6. Pneumococcal polysaccharide refers to the capsule that surrounds the bacterium *Streptococcus pneumoniae.*
7. Polysaccharides refer to antigens that are T independent antigens.
8. Somatic recombination refers to the expression of unique B cell receptors in which DNA is rearranged.
9. B cell receptor encoding refers to the set of events that leads to the expression of many different B cell receptors first elucidated in Tonegawa's laboratory in 1978. Heterodimers CD79a/b (associated with the membrane-bound antibody) transmit a message to signaling cascades that impact on the nucleus affecting transcription leading to the production of proteins, and eventually division of the cell leading to clones with the same specificity .
10. CD 19 is a molecule that regulates B cell development, activation, and differentiation.
11. CD20 is an ion channel expressed on pre-B and B cells.
12. Recombinases are special enzymes performing tasks of cutting and pasting DNA.
13. CD40 and CD40L refers to key interactions occurring between B cells and T cells along with cytokines that make up the costimulatory signal necessary for B cells to switch isotypes and form memory cells. CD 40 is a molecule on B cells, and CD40L is a molecule on T cells.

True or False

1. True
2. True
3. False
4. True
5. True

Fill in the Blank

1. memory cells
2. somatic recombination
3. recombinases
4. Monomeric IgM
5. anergic

Multiple Choice

1. c
2. a
3. d
4. b
5. b

Critical Thinking 1

1. Specificity refers to a clone of B cells all having the same receptor recognizing the same antigen. B cells may express 10 to the tenth power different B cell clones with different B cell receptors, and B cells may have as many as 25,000 antibodies (B cell receptors) on their cell surface, so while Tom is thinking about what may work for the individual having an immune response, "what works or not" does not convey the complexity of the situation.
2. Kim can offer more of the story on specificity by talking about the chemistry and genetics involved. She can mention Tonegawa's work on receptor encoding, which covers a lot of the chemistry and genetics. For the full story, Kim would mention somatic recombination to get the unique receptors in the first place with discussion of the "V," "D," and "J" segments. Tolerance induction would be a good thing to talk about, too, since without it there will be self-reactive IgM (B cell receptors).
3. B cells may express as many as 25,000 antibodies (B cell receptors) on their cell surface. The B cell acquires its receptor during the maturation process in the bone marrow.

Critical Thinking 2

1. Random selection of V, (D), and J segments in the construction of variable regions of the light and heavy chains leads inevitably to B cell receptors whose variable regions recognize self; these are autoreactive!
2. Normally these autoreactive receptors are deleted, or inactivated in the bone marrow during immature B cell stage of development. Immature B cells with the self-reactive IgM (B cell receptor) that bind self-antigens become unresponsive (anergic) to further stimulation or they die in a process known as tolerance induction.
3. Tolerance induction must not be active triggering anergy or apoptosis in self-reactive immature B cells for autoimmune responses to be prevalent. Bone marrow must be healthy, proper T cell stimulation for necessary cytokines for specific memory cells, et cetera must all be normal. A healthy immune system will not allow autoreactive responses.

Case Study

1. When the body encounters a "bug," the immune response depends on the site of antigen entry: if it enters the blood, the spleen will be the first contact; if it enters via the skin, the cutaneous immune system or draining lymph node will produce the mediate response; and if the bug comes into the body through any mucosal surface, then mucosal-associated lymphatic tissue (MALT) respond first. Whenever and wherever B cells do encounter antigens, however, there is interaction via receptors and the complexes are internalized, forming an endosome. Degraded antigen fragments are bound to MHC proteins (type II) and then expressing the antigen fragment/MHC complex on the B

cell surface. This complex interacts with a T cell for the next phase of B cell activation. Activated B cells, having received appropriate signals from T cells, undergo proliferation known as clonal expansion. The initial encounter is termed the primary immune response.

2. Secondary immune responses are those in which memory cells (with higher avidity for the antigen than the original B cell clone from the primary response due to affinity maturation or somatic mutation) are activated following encounter with the antigen. More rapid increases in IgG will be observed in secondary immune responses. Lag time is quicker in secondary responses as well as a larger response.

3. Interactions between B cells and T cells are primarily important in primary immune responses, as well as B cell clonal expansion after activation and the proliferation of plasma cells expressing the specific antibody. (There are T cell independent antigens, however, which induce B cell activation without T cell help like polysaccharides; memory cells are dependent on signals derived from T cells, however, so negligible if any isotype switching and memory cell formation occurs.)

CHAPTER 6

Matching

1. m
2. p
3. t
4. h
5. u
6. r
7. q
8. a
9. k
10. e
11. s
12. o
13. f
14. j
15. i
16. g
17. n
18. c
19. d
20. l
21. b

Definitions

1. MHC refers to the major histocompatibility complex, a gene region located in chromosome 6 in humans that encodes classes of antigen-presenting molecules.
2. Class I MHC can be identified on all human nucleated cells, and these molecules bind to antigen fragments within the cell and then the complex is displayed on the surface of infected cells.
3. MLR refers to mixed lymphocyte reaction, a laboratory technique used to determine if one set of T cells will be activated when they interact with class II MHC proteins present on another individual's cells.

4. Linkage disequilibrium refers to two genes inherited together in higher frequency than would be predicted by chance.
5. GvHD refers to graft versus host disease that is a rejection process in which the graft rejects all the recipient tissues.
6. RFLP refers to restriction fragment length polymorphism that is a technique in which enzymes are used to cleave genomic DNA and can be used to assess compatibility for transplantation.
7. PCR refers to polymerase chain reaction that is an automated, simple, rapid, *in vitro* technique allowing direct amplification of a particular DNA sequence in the presence of primers that border the gene of interest.
8. TAP proteins are transporters in antigen processing.
9. Endosomes are cytosolic vesicles.
10. Class II MHC refers to encoding for proteins that regulate the immune response in that, in their absence, helper T cells cannot be activated. Almost all aspects of host defense require helper T cell-derived molecules.
11. Genotype refers to the sum of haplotypes in a human; the total alleles inherited from both parents.
12. Polymorphic refers to having many forms.
13. Allelic refers to variant forms of a specific gene.

True or False

1. True
2. False
3. False
4. True
5. True

Fill in the Blank

1. progression
2. cross-reactive
3. linkage disequilibrium
4. isograft
5. graft versus host disease

Multiple Choice

1. b
2. c
3. d
4. c

Critical Thinking 1

1. Sarah's chart supporting genetic predisposition for MHC genes and disease would have results of epidemiological studies showing that the HLA alleles that an individual inherits may predispose that individual to certain diseases. Examples would include the HLA-B27 allele that is tied to a risk for ankylosing spondylitis, an inflammatory disorder and rheumatoid arthritis that occurs primarily in individuals who carry the HLA-DR4 allele. Sarah would use Table 6.1 for more examples. (Relative risks involve cross-reactivity, receptors, linkage disequilibrium, determinant selection, tolerance, and molecular mimicry.)
2. Kim wants a more balanced view of all research and she would bring up the risk factors and the fact that some individuals contract the diseases without benefit of the allele correlated with them.

3. The debate about association with disease and alleles is useful in determining the apparent risks, and may target individuals who might choose appropriate prophylactic therapy if available. If there is no therapy available for a specific predisposition, it becomes a no-win situation, but even then research is advancing, there is always hope, and there will always be those who choose to know rather than be ignorant of their future.

Critical Thinking 2

1. The major difference between a nursing view and an immunological view concerning burns and grafts is academic versus clinical. Grafting involves the transplantation issue and genetic disparity: isografts have no genetic difference, allografts are made between members of the same species, and xenografts are grafts between different species. Graft rejection is of concern to the immunology student who has looked at hyperacute, acute or chronic rejections, and graft versus host disease. The nursing student is more concerned with the initial survival of the patient before a graft can even be contemplated, and is much more concerned about fluid loss and secondary infection since the burn has breached the first line of immune defense.
2. Once the burn patient has been stabilized, the differences between immunology students and nursing students disappear as both are then concerned about tissue typing and tissue matching to prescreen recipients and potential donors to ensure the best possible genetic match to minimize the likelihood of rejection.
3. The most vigorous rejection episodes occur in acute rejection, especially hyperacute that occurs minutes to hours after engraftment. Grafts can be promoted via therapies that target the T cells. (Acute rejection is a T cell-mediated event.) Immunosuppressive drugs include cyclosporin A, FK506, prednisone, and antibodies targeting specific cell surface molecules.

Case Study

1. A paternity suit would include histocompatibility testing for exclusion, because if the child does not express any of the same HLA alleles as the male being tested, the paternity can be excluded. These tests would be tissue matching tests involving restriction fragment length polymorphism and polymerase chain reaction; tissue typing would include determining HLA alleles expressed on the leukocytes through serological tests. A unique sequence of nucleic acid patterns (RFLPs) is inherited and can be visualized with almost 100% accuracy of genetic relatedness by electrophoresis.
2. Exclusion is demonstrated by the HLA alleles, but DNA analysis (DNA "fingerprinting") is most accurate for paternity.
3. The science concerns the inheritance of alleles determined by paternity.

CHAPTER 7

Matching

1. h
2. t
3. l
4. a
5. o
6. c
7. j
8. e

9. r
10. n
11. u
12. b
13. s
14. i
15. q
16. f
17. d
18. p
19. k
20. g
21. m

Definitions

1. AIDS refers to acquired immunodeficiency disease syndrome in which the ratio of CD4+ T cells and CD8+ T cells is diagnostic.
2. T cells are cells that contribute to all aspects of immunity; also known as T lymphocytes.
3. TCR refers to T cell receptor that interacts with the MHC complexes on the cell surface.
4. T cell maturation refers to the process that the progenitor T cell arriving to the thymus undergoes to become able to act in host defense.
5. Thymocyte refers to developing T cells in the thymus.
6. Somatic recombination refers to the process by which gene segments are rearranged.
7. Recombinases are special enzymes that aid in the cutting and pasting of DNA.
8. Chimeric gene refers to one constructed by randomly selecting one "V" segment, one "D" segment, and one "J" segment of the many available.
9. T cell activation refers to the differentiation process of T cells during an immune response based upon signals received by Thp cells.
10. Interferon gamma refers to a cytokine secreted by activated natural killer cells and Th1 cells.
11. Memory cells are cells that ensure that the immune system can readily respond to subsequent infections by the same organism that triggered differentiation of their precursor (Thp).
12. Perforin refers to lytic granules secreted by the CTL in a polarized fashion to the targeted infected cells.
13. Isolation of T cells refers to the use of magnetic beads to which antibodies specific for cell surface markers are attached. Positive selection refers to the antibody on the magnet being specific for a molecule on the T cell, whereas in negative selection a number of different antibodies specific for markers on non T cells are attached to the magnetic beads

True or False

1. True
2. False
3. False
4. False
5. True

Fill in the Blank

1. major histocompatibility complex
2. clone
3. repertoire

4. maturation
5. thymocyte

Multiple Choice

1. b
2. e
3. a
4. e

Critical Thinking 1

1. General things to say about naïve CD4 T cell activation include that it must take place as an initial encounter with an antigen in a secondary lymphoid tissue, which constitutes a primary immune response, and that activation only occurs if the appropriate costimulatory signals are present. Naïve here only means having not yet encountered an antigen, not that it cannot participate in host defense. The differentiation from thymocyte to CD4+ T cell or CD8+ T cell has already occurred within the thymus.
2. The two sorts of cytokines that mediate the immune process are Type 1 cytokines secreted by Th1 cells (supporting host defenses in which macrophages, natural killer cells, and cytotoxic T cells are effectors), and Type 2 cytokines secreted by Th2 cells (inducing C cell activation and differentiation to plasma cells).
3. A naïve CD4+ T cell can become either a Th1 or Th2 cell depending on the pattern of cytokines in the local microenvironment, the concentration of antigen, and the type of antigen-presenting cell. When interferon gamma is predominant in the microenvironment, the naïve T helper cell will preferentially differentiate into Th 1 cells, while if interleukin 4 (IL-4) predominates, the naïve T helper cell will preferentially develop into Th 2 cells.

Critical Thinking 2

1. Tom and Sarah have overheard the nursing student's remark that the body just "learns how to fight off the infectious agent more effectively" concerning the difference between immune system responses initially to antigen and subsequent responses, and they reply by saying that while there is a more effective secondary response in terms of antibody titer and rapidity of response there are lots of things the nursing student needs to understand. One of those things being that memory cells are a crucial part of this subsequent immune response beginning immediately instead of having to depend on the differentiation of a pCTL to a CTL for example.
2. Differences between CD4+ and CD8+ T cells in this process include that memory CD4+ T cells can be activated at the site of infection while CD8+ cytotoxic cell clones recirculate to perform an immunosurveillance role. Naïve CD8+ T cells do not need to encounter antigen in a secondary lymphoid tissue in contrast to CD4+ T cells.
3. Time differences in initial and subsequent encounters with an infectious agent are the following: initial differentiation of naïve cells to their mature counterpart is around 7 days, whereas memory cells incite a response in 1 to 2 days. The time difference is accounted for by the initial time to differentiate the naïve cells.

CHAPTER 8

Matching

1. n
2. t
3. g
4. a
5. s
6. o
7. j
8. l
9. d
10. h
11. f
12. i
13. k
14. e
15. q
16. b
17. r
18. m
19. p
20. c

Definitions

1. Complement refers to a system of numerous proteins playing an important role in host defense.
2. Classical pathway refers to activation of complement that requires antibody.
3. Alternative pathway refers to activation of complement not requiring antibody.
4. Cascade refers to complement activation because the numerous proteins of the complement system are sequentially activated.
5. Complement fixation refers to the first component of complement when C1 binds with IgM or IgG bound to a bacterial cell's surface.
6. Anaphylatoxins are small molecules binding to receptors present on mast cells and basophils.
7. MAC refers to membrane attack complex that is a transmembrane channel allowing a rapid influx of ions into the bacterial cell.
8. Properdin is a regulatory protein in the alternative pathway.
9. Common pathway refers to a segment of the activation pathway containing the membrane attack complex; also called the terminal pathway.
10. Complement receptors are Type 1 (CR1) regulatory protein, Type 2 (CR2) receptor for inactivated C3b, Type 3 (CR3) receptor for iC3b, and others.
11. Degranulation refers to release of inflammatory mediators including histamine from anaphylatoxin interaction with receptors on mast cells and basophils.
12. Chemokines are molecules attracting cells to certain sites and playing an important role in the inflammatory response.
13. Bradykinin is a small peptide produced when kallikrein cleaves kininogen; it induces vascular permeability.

True or False

1. True
2. False
3. True
4. True

Fill in the Blank

1. Complement
2. classical
3. alternative
4. C1 INH, C4bp, DAF, CR1, CD59, HRF
5. properdin

Multiple Choice

1. e
2. b
3. d
4. d

Critical Thinking 1

1. The regulatory proteins for complement include C1 inhibitor, C4 binding protein, delay accelerating factor, anaphylatoxin inhibitor, vitronectin, properdin, et cetera. They are essentially for inhibition, for example, inhibition of complement activation or inhibition of MAC formation. They affect complement by accelerating dissociation of convertases, or binding or cleaving molecules to effect inhibition of MAC or anaphylatoxins, et cetera. Autologous cells refer to self-cells as opposed to xenograft cells from another species (e.g., porcine).
2. The two complement pathways are classical (activation requiring antibody) and alternative (activation not requiring antibody). They both share a terminal pathway leading to a membrane attack complex. Students in immunology may be confused about the complement pathways because of all the various regulatory proteins and their complexity, numbers of complement proteins, and figuring out similarities and differences.
3. Complement is regulated by many different proteins that must be activated by amplification. This regulation and amplification does shed some light on the complexity of complement (for example, because the activation of the classical pathway of complement is amplified when it recruits the alternative pathway of complement via production of C3b). Antibody is not necessary for activation of the alternative pathway and can function without the adaptive immune system, and aggregated IgA can activate the alternative pathway in a non-specific manner.

Critical Thinking 2

1. Examples of WBCs exiting the blood vessels to enter infected areas include neutrophils and monocytes differentiating into macrophages. They exit the vascular compartment attracted via chemotaxis to tissue trauma.
2. Chemokines are molecules/chemicals attracting macrophages and neutrophils to certain sites. Histamine (released by the degranulation of mast cells and basophils after anaphylatoxins like C3a, C4a, and C5a bind to their cognate receptors) is one of the agents inducing an increase in vascular permeability allowing the neutrophils, for example, to emigrate via diapedesis into inflammatory sites.

3. In the spleen and liver, RBCs with CR1 receptors on them, like neutrophils, are stripped of their immune complexes by macrophages.

Case Study

1. From an immunological point of view, recurrent gonorrhea, meningitis, angioedema, and PNH are deficiencies in complement proteins and associated disorders.
2. You explain these disorders to your nursing friend by saying that a deficiency in C1-INH leads to angioedema, a deficiency of C2 and C4 leads to immune complex disorders, a deficiency of C3 leads to pyrogenic infections with encapsulated bacteria, deficiencies of C5, 6, 7, 8, 9 result in recurrent infections with *Neisseria sp.*, and a deficiency of GPI linkages (DAF and CD59) results in paroxysmal nocturnal hemoglobinuria.
3. The following tests/assays may be used to screen for these disorders: first, a test is made to look for deficiencies causing an overall reduction in complement activation (CH50 and AH50 which measure overall complement activity of the classical and the alternative complement pathways respectively); second, tests for individual components are made to determine which one(s) are defective (radial immunodiffusion test or rate nephelometry).

CHAPTER 9

Matching

1. t
2. d
3. m
4. s
5. o
6. u
7. r
8. e
9. p
10. a
11. f
12. c
13. b
14. i
15. g
16. n
17. k
18. h
19. j
20. l
21. q

Definitions

1. MALT refers to mucosa associated lymphoid tissues.
2. Histamine is released from the degranulation of mast cells and basophils.
3. Bradykinin is a small peptide that is a potent molecule acting on endothelial cells to cause an increase in vascular permeability.

4. Osmotic lysis refers to what happens to bacteria following insertion of the membrane attack complex.
5. Anaphylatoxins are small molecules (C3a and C5a) binding to receptors present on mast cells and basophils.
6. Interleukin-1 and TNF are cytokines secreted by activated macrophages acting locally on the endothelial cells.
7. Chemotactic refers to molecules that attract neutrophils and monocytes to the infection site.
8. Diapedesis is the process by which neutrophils and monocytes bind to the endothelium and secrete enzymes degrading the basement membrane between the endothelial cells allowing neutrophils to squeeze into the infection site.
9. Thp cells are T helper precursor cells or naïve CD4+ T cells.
10. Interferon gamma is a Type 1 cytokine inducing monocytes to differentiate to macrophages.
11. *Mycobacterium tuberculosis* is the causative agent of tuberculosis.
12. Proteasome is a large multimeric complex consisting of several proteases.
13. Ubiquitin is a small highly conserved protein in all cell's cytoplasm and nuclei that targets proteins for proteasome degradation by covalently binding to them.

True or False

1. False
2. False
3. True
4. False
5. True

Fill in the Blank

1. phagosome
2. phagocytosis
3. histamine
4. MHC
5. B cells

Multiple Choice

1. c
2. d
3. e
4. c

Critical Thinking Exercise

1. The molecules Tom is referring to with IL-1 and TNF are cytokines. The part of the body that they act upon is the hypothalamus and they induce fever.
2. Other molecules in this class of molecules are Type 1 (interferon gamma) and Type 2 cytokines. The effects of cytokines are varied from inducing monocyte differentiation to macrophages, activating vascular endothelial cells to become more adhesive, and really regulating almost every aspect of immunity.
3. Sarah explains that fever is such a part of infection because (from a human anatomy and physiology point of view) the elevated body temperature kills some infectious agents and it also accelerates the healing processes of the body (speeding up immune responses) within limits of extreme elevation and extreme duration.

Case Study

1. The immunology students mention that phagocytosis is one of the immune system's methods of targeting microbes outside of cells. Tissue macrophages secrete many proteins causing inflammation, chemotactic molecules, cytokines (inducing fever and altering the differentiation of CD4+ Thp cells to Th1 cells), and inducing expression of heat shock proteins in the liver. Cells get to where they need to be by diapedesis.
2. The cells that are phagocytic include neutrophils and macrophages.
3. Phagocytes are different structurally and functionally, for example, eosinophils, (that target helminths) neutrophils (most prevalent granular leukocyte) and tissue macrophages (differentiated from monocytes).

CHAPTER 10

Matching

1. u
2. k
3. a
4. m
5. p
6. r
7. d
8. g
9. b
10. t
11. i
12. s
13. j
14. q
15. c
16. l
17. e
18. f
19. n
20. h
21. o

Definitions

1. A monochromator is a wave selector in a spectrophotometer.
2. A filter is a device that transmits some wavelengths of monochromatic light and absorbs all others.
3. A photomultiplier tube is a detector used in spectrophotometers that converts light into electrical signals.
4. A luminometer is a device that measures amounts of chemiluminescence.
5. Wavelength is a function of the energy contained in electromagnetic phenomena like gamma radiation, fluorescence, and visible light.
6. Quenching refers to decreasing the fluorescent intensity.

7. A flow cytometer is an instrument that uses a laser to quantitate components or structural features of cells by optical means, displaying the data graphically.
8. AIDS is acquired immunodeficiency syndrome caused by HIV.
9. Direct labeling refers to a cell surface molecule on the antibody directly interacting with the target molecule.
10. Indirect labeling refers to a cell surface molecule on a secondary antibody targeting the Fc region of antibodies bound to the cell.
11. ELISA refers to enzyme linked immunoabsorbent assay.
12. Fluorescent microscopes are instruments used to detect cell surface molecules or molecules within tissues.
13. VDRL refers to venereal diseases research laboratory.

True or False

1. True
2. True
3. False
4. False
5. True

Fill in the Blank

1. Gamma ray emission, fluorescence, and chemiluminescence
2. alkaline phosphatase
3. wave selector
4. monochromator
5. Chemiluminescence

Multiple Choice

1. a
2. c
3. e
4. d

Critical Thinking Exercise

1. Tom and Sarah explain nephelometry to Kim by defining it as the process of measuring the amount of light scattering caused by immune complexes. Spectrophotometry monitors the amount of a given wavelength of light entering a solution and the amount that is transmitted.
2. Advantages of nephelometry are speed and precision, but the disadvantage is the cost of instrumentation.
3. The presence of dust, scratched/dirty cuvettes, and contaminated reagents all adversely affect the precision of nephelometry, so meticulous care must be used when filtering reagents and selecting cuvettes. Turbidimetry is the process of measuring of the amount of light absorbed by the immune complexes (versus measuring the light scattered by these complexes in nephelometry approaches).

CHAPTER 11

Matching

1. h
2. m
3. p
4. a
5. c
6. j
7. e
8. n
9. l
10. b
11. g
12. i
13. f
14. o
15. k
16. d

Definitions

1. Alkaline phosphatase is an enzyme usually isolated from calf intestine used as an indirect indicator label.
2. Fluorescence refers to molecules (fluorochromes) that absorb light and become transiently excited; when the excited molecule returns to a more stable state, most of the energy is then emitted as visible light.
3. Horseradish peroxidase is an enzyme derived from plants that is used as an indirect indicator label.
4. Glutaraldehyde is a bifunctional reagent covalently cross-linking two amino acids.
5. Biotinylated antibody refers to the preparatory step in the biotin-streptavidin system in which biotin is coupled to antibody (biotin in DMSO incubated with antibody or antigen for one hour).
6. Standard curve refers to calibration curve samples performed under conditions identical to those of the patient's; for many clinical tests it is important to know the actual concentration of antigen or antibody in the biological sample and interpolate those measures onto a standard curve.
7. Serial dilution refers to the repetitive dilution of a sample by the same amount.
8. Competitive assays refer to tests in which labeled and non-labeled antigen compete for the same sites on an antibody.
9. Non-competitive assays refer to tests in which the antigen and antibody are allowed to interact without intended competition from other molecules.
10. RIA refers to radiolabeled immunoassay which is a test using radioactive isotopes as labels to detect antigen in a biological sample.
11. FIA refers to fluorochrome immunoassay, which is a test using fluorochromes as indicators.
12. ELISA refers to enzyme linked immunoabsorbent assay, which is a non-competitive assay to detect antigen or antibody in a biological sample.
13. FPIA refers to fluorescent polarization immunoassay, which is a non-classic, competitive immunoassay used to detect illegal and therapeutic drugs.

True or False

1. True
2. False
3. False
4. False
5. True

Fill in the Blank

1. (strept)avidin
2. fluorescence
3. spectrophotometer
4. standard curve
5. Serial dilution

Multiple Choice

1. a
2. b
3. d
4. c

Critical Thinking Exercise

1. The classical competitive immunoassay, RIA, is used to measure hormones and neurotransmitters.
2. The biological sample contains the antigen whose concentration is measured. Labeled and unlabeled antigen (from the patient sample) compete for binding to an antibody with an unknown specificity. The antibody needs to have the same avidity for both labeled and non-labeled antigen since there are limited binding sites on the antibody. The indicator label is either radioisotope or fluorochrome. The goal is to see if antigen-X is in a patient sample, and labeled antigen-X and anti-X antibodies are bought commercially. Anti-X antibodies are incubated with a protein A coated solid phase (microtiter plate) followed by washing to remove unbound antibodies. Non-specific binding sites are blocked by incubating the solid phase with albumin or gelatin, followed by washing to remove unbound protein. The biological sample and the commercially obtained antigen-X (with a known concentration) are added simultaneously to the plate in which antibody is bound. The antigens compete, and washing removes unbound antigen-X. Amount of labeled antigen-X in the wash, and amount bound to antibody is then measured appropriately for whichever label.
3. Other competitive immunoassays in this category include EMIT and FPIA.

Case Study

1. Non-competitive immunoassays are tests in which antigen and antibody are allowed to interact without any intentional introduction of competing molecules.
2. The protocol for these assays detects antigen in a biological sample. In ELISA, specific antibody, which is bound to a solid phase, is allowed to bind antigen in a biological sample without any impediment. Non-competitive immunoassays are either indirect (detect antibody in biological sample) or antibody sandwich approach to detect antigen. It is important to block the non-specific binding sites on the solid phase. In the antibody sandwich technique, non-labeled antibody of known specificity (anti-X antibodies) are bound to solid phase, and then washed to remove unbound antibody. Non-specific binding sites on solid phase are blocked by incubation with albumin or gelatin, and then washed. Sample is incubated with bound antibody, and then washed to remove

unbound material. A labeled anti-antigen X antibody is incubated with the immunocomplexes. Labeled anti-antigen X antibody will bind to the antigen. Detection depends on indicator label. If label is an enzyme, a substrate is added (and determines instrumentation type for detection). If antigen is bound to two antibodies, one on solid phase, one with indicator label, the test is done with antigens of the size to allow it.

CHAPTER 12

Matching

1. k
2. r
3. u
4. n
5. c
6. p
7. s
8. l
9. g
10. q
11. t
12. a
13. h
14. i
15. f
16. j
17. m
18. b
19. o
20. d
21. e

Definitions

1. Hydrogen bonds are chemical bonds in which a hydrogen atom on one molecule is attracted to an atom on another molecule.
2. Ionic bonds are bonds forming between oppositely charged ionic groups on two protein side chains.
3. Van der Waals forces are interactions between electron clouds present around antibodies and antigens.
4. Affinity is the bond strength between an epitope and its corresponding complementary site with the Fab region of the antibody.
5. Avidity is the overall strength of the entire antibody interaction with antigen.
6. Precipitation is a phase change in which soluble reactants form an insoluble product.
7. Multivalent antigens have more than one epitope.
8. Univalent antigens have only one epitope.
9. Flocculation is natural clumping.

10. Precipitin curve refers to a graphic representation of precipitin reactions occurring under particular experimental conditions.
11. The equivalence point is the point at which the maximal possible precipitant forms.
12. Immunodiffusion is a phenomenon referring to the diffusion of antigen and/or antibodies.

True or False

1. False
2. False
3. True
4. True
5. False

Fill in the Blank

1. Cross-linking
2. Multivalent
3. immunoprecipitation
4. Precipitation curve
5. equivalence point

Multiple Choice

1. c
2. e
3. d
4. d

Critical Thinking Exercise

1. Tom is talking about hydrogen and ionic bonds and Van der Waals forces.
2. Sarah could explain that formation of antibody/antigen complexes is the result of these non-covalent, intermolecular interactions between antigen and Fab region of an antibody.
3. Primary reactions are the result of the non-covalent, intermolecular interactions, while secondary reactions occur as a result of the primary antibody/antigen interactions. Precipitation is an example of the secondary reaction.

Case Study

1. Tom has learned that apoproteins are the protein components of lipoproteins that are plasma proteins that are transporters of cholesterol and triacylglycerol. Lipoproteins can be measured by radial immunodiffusion.
2. Single radial immunodiffusion is a technique used to determine quantitatively the antigen concentration in a solution. Antibody is in the gel and the antigen is the mobile reagent. Formation, dissolution, and formation of the precipitin band is in a radial pattern, and the endpoint is a precipitin ring instead of a band.
3. Statin refers to a type of pharmaceutical that prevents the liver from making cholesterol by interfering with a particular enzyme necessary for its synthesis. An example of a statin is Lipitor™. Tom's uncle is most probably on a diet low in cholesterol and saturated fats and triglycerides.

CHAPTER 13

Matching

1. l
2. g
3. p
4. a
5. j
6. k
7. c
8. n
9. b
10. e
11. o
12. f
13. i
14. m
15. d
16. h

Definitions

1. Electrophoresis is a technique in which molecules separate by charge when an electric field is applied.
2. Non-soluble support media refer to media that constrain movement of molecules, and are used now for separation of biological molecules.
3. Isoelectric point is that pH in which positive charges on a protein balance the negative.
4. Electro-osmosis refers to the net flow of hydrated ions in one direction in an applied electric field ; also known as endo-osmosis.
5. Agar is a polysaccharide mixture of agarose and agaropectin.
6. Agarose is a linear polysaccharide binding to ions in a buffer when the pH is neutral.
7. Cellulose acetate is a support medium made by treating cellulose with acetic anhydride.
8. Zone electrophoresis is a technique in which proteins and nucleic acids are separated and form separate bands or zones.
9. Classic immunoelectrophoresis is a two-stage process with both electrophoretic separation of proteins and diffusion.
10. Crossed immunoelectrophoresis is a two-stage process with both electrophoretic separation of proteins followed by electrophoresis at a 90-degree angle to the first step; also called two-dimensional immunoelectrophoresis (2D-IEF).
11. Immunofixation is a two-stage process with electrophoretic separation of proteins followed with a second stage immunoprecipitation.
12. Counter immunoelectrophoresis is a method used to screen biological samples for presence of bacterial and viral antigens.
13. Rocket immunoelectrophoresis is a one-stage technique combining electrophoresis and antigen migration into an antibody containing gel.

True or False

1. False
2. False
3. True
4. True
5. True

Fill in the Blank

1. Electro-osmosis (endo-osmosis)
2. Agar
3. Cellulose acetate
4. Zone electrophoresis
5. densitometer

Multiple Choice

1. a
2. e
3. d
4. c

Critical Thinking Exercise

1. Electrophoresis is a technique in which molecules are separated on charge in an applied electric field. It could be used to identify antigens on pathogens (bacterial, fungi, viruses in biological fluids).
2. Counter and immunofixation immunoelectrophoresis could be useful respectively in diagnoses of hepatitis B antigen and monitoring serum monoclonal proteins like in myeloma.
3. Counter immunoelectrophoresis is the electrophoretically-induced migration of proteins (antigens) toward the anode and the antibody, while antibody is induced to migrate toward the cathode and the proteins (antigen); precipitin band forms where complexes form, and immunoprecipitate may be stained with a protein dye. Immunofixation electrophoresis is the electrophoretic separation of proteins in biological sample, and then introduction of antibody on top of each electrophoretic migration track; precipitin band occurs when overlaid antibody diffuses into the gel and forms complexes with antigen and are trapped in the gel matrix. The surprise is because these tests are complicated with requisites of voltage, running temperatures, and prohibitive costs often not available in third world countries.

CHAPTER 14

Matching

1. l
2. f
3 q
4. k
5. o
6. m
7. d

8. a
9. j
10. r
11. h
12. n
13. b
14. p
15. c
16. g
17. e
18. i

Definitions

1. Agglutination is the clumping and sedimentation of particulate antigen/antibody complexes.
2. Lattice formation is the result of antibody interactions with multivalent antigens.
3. Antibody titer is the highest dilution of a biological sample that still results in agglutination.
4. Zone of equivalence refers to the region in a serum sample where maximal agglutination occurs between prozone and post zone.
5. Electrolytes refer to salts or ions, which are required for agglutination reactions to occur.
6. Slide test is a qualitative test used to screen large numbers of sera.
7. Microtiter plates are used for serial dilutions, as in determining serum antibody titer; microtiter plates are 96 well plates that are essentially very small tubes.
8. Direct agglutination is a test in which the antigen is an intrinsic component of the particle; used to ascertain whether antibody specific for antigen is in biological fluids.
9. Indirect agglutination is a reaction in which the antigen has been affixed or absorbed to the particle surface.
10. HCG refers to human chorionic gonadotrophin; test confirming pregnancy.
11. Sol particle immunoassay is a test using antibodies or antigens to bind to colloidal particles.
12. Dispersal dye immunoassay is a test in which organic dye colloidal particles are used for agglutination immunoassay.
13. Zeta potential refers to the electrostatic potential made around erythrocytes in solution.

True or False

1. True
2. False
3. True
4. True
5. True

Fill in the Blank

1. agglutinins
2. Lattices
3. Antibody titer
4. zone of equivalence
5. Buffers

Multiple Choice

1. c
2. b
3. a
4. e

Critical Thinking

1. Agglutination is simply the clumping together and sedimentation of particulate antigen/antibody complexes.
2. The factors affecting agglutination include buffer pH, relative concentration of antibody and antigen, location and concentration of epitopes (antigenic determinants) on the particle, electrostatic interactions between particles, electrolyte concentration, antibody isotype, and temperature.
3. Tests using agglutination include SPIA, DIA, IMPACT, hemagglutination (direct or indirect, reverse, viral), anti-globulins tests, and direct Coombs' test (direct or indirect).

CHAPTER 15

Matching

1. g
2. s
3. k
4. u
5. o
6. f
7. m
8. a
9. d
10. b
11. q
12. i
13. t
14. h
15. e
16. n
17. c
18. p
19. j
20. r
21. l

Definitions

1. Annealing refers to cooling a mixture allowing primers to bind with complementary regions.
2. Western blot is used to diagnose Lyme disease and confirm HIV infection.
3. Fragile-X syndrome is an inherited condition associated with mental retardation, long narrow face with prominent jaw and forehead (FMR-1 gene changes in repeated sequences and methylation on X chromosome).

4. Sickle cell disease is a genetic disorder caused by a single DNA mutation in the beta globin gene that leads to sickle cell anemia (due to red blood cells assuming sickle shape under reduced oxygen tension).
5. Methylation refers to chemical changes associated with fragile-X syndrome in which methyl groups are added at critical sites along the FMR-1 gene on the X chromosome.
6. Southern blot detects specific DNA sequences (RFLP fragments) separated by agarose gel electrophoresis by size and transferred to nitrocellulose or a nylon membrane.
7. Nucleic acids are DNA and RNA; macromolecular polymers composed of nucleotide monomers (sugar, phosphate residue, base).
8. Ribose is a pentose sugar specific for RNA.
9. Uracil is a pyrimidine base specific for RNA.
10. The term hnRNA refers to heterogeneous RNA that includes non-coding (intron) regions that are spliced in conversion to mRNA.
11. Transcription is the copying of the DNA triplet code to the RNA triplet codon.
12. Processing/splicing refers to the removal or deletion of introns in the hnRNA creating mRNA in eukaryotes.
13. Translation is the process in which the mRNA codon and its nucleotide base sequence are used to create the amino acid sequence in prospective proteins coded for by the DNA in the first place.

True or False

1. True
2. False
3. False
4. True
5. False

Fill in the Blank

1. DNA
2. Nucleic acids
3. bases
4. double helix
5. complementary

Multiple Choice

1. d
2. e
3. a
4. e

Critical Thinking Exercise

1. In transcription from DNA to hnRNA and ultimately to mRNA in eukaryotes, the base uracil substitutes complementarily with adenine instead of thymine.
2. The differences between the nucleic acids RNA and DNA are fundamentally what Tom needs to understand.
3. DNA is a double-stranded helix that has a different pentose sugar (deoxyribose), and has the bases A, T, C, and G; whereas RNA is single-stranded, has ribose as its sugar in the nucleotide, and uses U, A, C, and G as its bases. Triplet codes are found on DNA that are transcribed to RNA codons, which translate into amino acid sequences, so functionally they are very different in the role they play in ultimately creating the proteins.

Case Study

1. Restriction enzymes (from bacteria) cleave DNA into fragments at specific nucleotide sequence sites.
2. They are essential to the famous DNA fingerprinting technique for example, which cleaves RFLPs unique to each individual except identical twins.
3. Restriction endonucleases are another name. In nature, bacteria defend themselves against viral phages by fragmenting their nucleic acids with restriction enzymes.

CHAPTER 16

Matching

1. f
2. s
3. k
4. r
5. a
6. u
7. c
8. o
9. h
10. q
11. p
12. m
13. d
14. j
15. b
16. e
17. l
18. t
19. i
20. n
21. g

Definitions

1. CCR5 refers to a macrophage receptor that *T. pallidum* or its lipoproteins induce.
2. Granulomatous refers to accumulations of modified macrophages and connective tissue; said of lesions associated with late benign syphilis.
3. Cardiolipin is part of treponemal lipids.
4. Delayed type hypersensitivity is a response to bacterial invasion; macrophages are activated whose cytotoxic potential is improved by Type 1 cytokines secreted by CD4+ T cells.
5. Seroconverted refers to antibodies in the blood.
6. Reagin antibodies refer to non-treponemal antibodies.
7. TPI refers to *T. pallidum* immobilization test.
8. Western blotting is a technique in which solubilized or recombinant *T. pallidum* antigens, electrophoretically separated and transferred to nitrocellulose or nylon membrane, are tested for anti-treponemal antibodies.
9. Asymptomatic means presenting no symptoms.

10. Neonates are newborns.
11. Opthalmia neonatorum refers to infections present in the eyes of newborns.
12. Secretory IgA is the predominant antibody in mucosal immunity.
13. The term, energy parasites, refers to reticulate bodies of *Chlamydiae* because they obtain their energy (ATP) from the host cell.

True or False

1. True
2. False
3. False
4. True

Fill in the Blank

1. Syphilis
2. congenital
3. chancre
4. reagin
5. factor H

Multiple Choice

1. c
2. a
3. b
4. b

Case Study

1. Syphilis. Male. Because of definitive symptoms for the male.
2. *Treponema pallidum*. It attacks abraded skin or mucous membranes during intimate contact. Antibodies are produced, as well as phagocytosis and complement activation.
3. No. It is an effective pathogen evading the immune system in ways not clearly understood at the present. Serological tests exist for diagnosis based on antigen/antibody interactions.

CHAPTER 17

Matching

1. m
2. t
3. q
4. p
5. s
6. i
7. a
8. o
9. u
10. d

11. r
12. f
13. c
14. e
15. b
16. h
17. n
18. k
19. g
20. l
21. j

Definitions

1. An acellular vaccine is one made with purified or recombinant proteins.
2. Atypical pneumonia is an infection presenting more viral than bacterial.
3. *Bordetella pertussis* is the causative agent of pertussis or whooping cough.
4. Catarrhal refers to the first stage of *B. pertussis* infection characterized by red eyes, runny nose, mild cough, sneezing, and fever.
5. Cilia are found on the epithelial cells of the respiratory tract to which bacteria attach.
6. Cold agglutinins are IgM antibodies reactive with glycophorin on RBCs.
7. Complement fixation is the reference method for serological testing, but it does not differentiate between IgG or IgM antibody titers.
8. Convalescent refers to the third stage of *B. pertussis* infection that lasts up to six months, in which the symptoms slowly attenuate.
9. GASD refers to Group A Streptococcal Direct test that is used for antigen detection of Group A *Streptococci*.
10. Filamentous hemagglutinin is a virulence factor for *B. pertussis*; an adhesin.
11. Lancefield refers to a classification system based on analysis of phenotypic characteristics of the *Streptococci*.
12. *Mycoplasma pneumoniae* is the causative agent of atypical pneumonia.
13. Walking pneumonia is atypical pneumonia, and so-called *walking* pneumonia because people with it continue to go to school or work even with the malaise.

True or False

1. False
2. True
3. True
4. False
5. False

Fill in the Blank

1. *Mycoplasma pneumoniae*
2. contagious
3. adhesive protein
4. PCR
5. digoxigenin (DIG-dUTP)

Multiple Choice

1. a
2. c
3. e
4. b

Critical Thinking Exercise

1. Streptococcal toxic shock syndrome.
2. *Streptococcus pyogenes* and especially group A strains that produce toxins referred to as streptococcal pyrogenic exotoxins (SPEs). There are four SPEs (A, B, C, and F) and these are virulence factors.
3. SPE toxins function as superantigens and stimulate a vast number of CD4+ T cells with unregulated release of cytokines, particularly Type I cytokines. Low blood pressure and shock are correlated with the vascular permeability inflammatory responses, and the hyaluronic acid allows for invasion into tissues and widespread dissemination of the bacterium. Lipoteichoic acid and M proteins enhance the pathogenicity of *S. pyogenes*, as well as streptokinase, C5a peptidase, and immunoglobulin binding proteins.

Case Study

1. Atypical or walking pneumonia caused by *Mycoplasma pneumoniae* is probably what Amy has contracted. Amy is presenting more like viral than bacterial, yet she is not bedridden even with all her malaise.
2. Bacteremia is rare, sputum is clear, and few deaths occur, but complications include IgA nephropathy, meningoencephalitis, anemia, and myocarditis.
3. Approaches to detect *M. pneumoniae* are of two types: detection of organism and antibody tests. Culture may be made of the organism from sputum or swabs as well as other body fluids, and specific antigen tests or molecular tests based on amplification techniques may be used for detection. Serological tests to diagnose *M. pneumoniae* infections by antibodies include complement fixation, indirect fluorescent test, cold agglutinin antibody titer, and enzyme linked immunosorbent assays (ELISA).

CHAPTER 18

Matching

1. e
2. u
3. l
4. q
5. a
6. o
7. h
8. c
9. s
10. b
11. t
12. f

13. n
14. d
15. j
16. i
17. p
18. k
19. m
20. g
21. r

Definitions

1. Anicteric leptospires refers to a self-limiting, relatively mild disease with low-grade fever caused by *Leptospira*.
2. Antigenic variation refers to sequences within genes constantly changing during an infection.
3. *Borrelia burgdorferi* is the spirochete bacterium that is the causative agent of Lyme disease.
4. Bull's eye appearance refers to the advancing, irregular bordered rash with a clear center as seen in 60 to 80% of individuals infected with *B. burgdorferi*.
5. The febrile agglutination test is also called Widal agglutination used to diagnose typhoid fever (q.v., below under definition for Widal agglutination).
6. FITC refers to fluorescein isothiocyanate used in the indirect fluorescent antibody assay.
7. Icteric leptospires is also called Weil's disease and is characterized by icterus (jaundice) and azotemia (urea in the blood).
8. The LEPTO Dri-Dot test is an agglutination test to detect antibodies specific for *Leptospira* antigens.
9. The LEPTO lateral flow test is a one-step colloidal gold immunoassay to detect antibodies for a *Leptospira* antigen.
10. Lyme disease is caused by *Borrelia burgdorferi* and is characterized by rash, fever, malaise, and headache.
11. *Rickettsia rickettsii* is the intracellular bacterium causing RMSF.
12. An example of a transmission blocking vaccine is LYMErix in which antibodies are produced to block the transmission of *B. burgdorferi* from tick to human.
13. Widal agglutination is a test developed to measure the presence of anti-O and anti-H antibodies in serum of patients with *Salmonella typhi*; also called the febrile agglutination test.

True or False

1. False
2. True
3. True
4. True
5. False

Fill in the Blank

1. *Borrelia burgdorferi*
2. ticks
3. peripheral facial palsy
4. Antigenic variation
5. virulence

Multiple Choice

1. e
2. b
3. a
4. b

Critical Thinking Exercise

1. Accidental hosts are hosts that are not the natural host. For example, humans are considered accidental hosts for *Leptospira interrogans* because the natural host for the organism is a wide range of domestic and wild animals. Zoonosis refers to an infectious disease in humans caused by an organism whose natural reservoir is non-human.
2. *Leptospira interrogans* is the organism, and leptospirosis is the disease.
3. Another example of a zoonosis is equine encephalitis virus in which song birds and mosquitoes and horses are all involved in the transmission of this serious disease. Multiple hosts could be a survival strategy for the organism or virus to exist when natural hosts were not possibly as available.

Case Study

1. Edith is showing signs of *Salmonella*-mediated gastroenteritis. Fluid and electrolyte replacement is crucial for severe diarrhea.
2. *Salmonella enteritidis* is the organism responsible.
3. Most serious complication of this infection is hemorrhage as a result of lesions in the intestinal wall where bacteria have attached and destroyed the M cells. Usually the infection is resolved in a week or less. Pathology is caused by colonizing the intestinal tract where they attach to M cells, are endocytosed, and are translocated to the lamina propria. From there the bacterium can be transported via lymph to the nodes and eventually to the blood. *Salmonella* possess endotoxins (e.g., lipopolysaccharides) responsible for much of the pathology. *Salmonella* resist destruction in the phagosome and so can proliferate.

CHAPTER 19

Matching

1. g
2. e
3. a
4. j
5. c
6. i
7. b
8. d
9. f
10. h

Definitions

1. Anti-HBs antibody reacts with three particles in sera from individuals infected with hepatitis B.
2. The six principal genotypes of HCV are referred to as clades.
3. The Dane particle is the intact, infectious hepatitis B virion.
4. E1 refers to an HCV membrane protein.
5. E2 refers to another HCV membrane protein that binds to a cell surface molecule (CD81) present on many human cells.
6. Until the development of a vaccine for hepatitis A, pooled human gamma globulins were used to passively immunize travelers to high-risk areas.
7. HAV is the causative agent of viral hepatitis A; single-stranded RNA within an icosahedral capsid.
8. HBV is the causative agent of viral hepatitis B; an enveloped DNA virus.
9. HCV is the causative agent of viral hepatitis C; an enveloped, single-stranded RNA; there are six principal genotypes or clades.

True or False

1. True
2. True
3. True
4. True
5. True

Fill in the Blank

1. clades
2. fecal-oral route
3. gamma globulins
4. Dane particle
5. Hepatitis B

Multiple Choice

1. e
2. b
3. a
4. b

Critical Thinking Exercise

1. The presumptive diagnosis is Hepatitis B virus (HBV) infection. Transmission is by direct contact with body fluids. High-risk individuals are IV drug users, sexual contact with infected individuals, and health care workers.
2. Main site of infection is liver parenchymal cells. Incubation time is variable ranging from six weeks to six months.
3. Tissue damage occurs due to the immunological response activated in response to HBV infection rather than direct toxicity to the liver cells.

CHAPTER 20

Matching

1. h
2. l
3. g
4. m
5. k
6. e
7. s
8. u
9. p
10. f
11. j
12. t
13. a
14. r
15. i
16. n
17. k
18. q
19. d
20. b
21. c

Definitions

1. Alkaline phosphatase is the label on murine anti-IgG antibodies to detect immune complexes in VIDAS.
2. Attenuvax is live attenuated measles virus used as a vaccine.
3. Chicken-pox is a varicella-zoster virus infection.
4. Congenital rubella syndrome refers to a serious condition in which a fetus receives rubella virus from the mother during the first trimester. The virus spreads to the fetus via the placenta and adversely affects development with possible outcomes such as cardiac anomalies, deafness, and mental retardation.
5. Fusion refers to a protein protruding from the viral envelope derived from the host cell plasma membrane, antigenically significant, and along with hemagglutinin, necessary to infect a cell.
6. German measles or rubella refers to a different infectious disease caused by a different virus from measles or rubeola, and is significant due to congenital rubella syndrome (q.v. above).
7. Hemagglutinin refers to a protein protruding from the viral envelope derived from the host cell plasma membrane, antigenically significant, and along with fusion protein, necessary to infect a cell.
8. Koplick's spots refer to spots on the mouth epithelium diagnostic for measles (rubeola or red measles).
9. Measles or red measles or rubeola is a highly contagious disease caused by the measles virus and characterized by photophobia, runny nose, fever, cough, and sneezing.
10. Mumps virus is the causative agent of the infectious disease known as mumps typically involving swelling of the parotid glands.

11. Reye's syndrome is a rare but very serious condition occurring in children recovering from vari-cella, especially those who ingested salicylates (e.g., aspirin) which is characterized by pathologies like encephalitis.
12. Varicella is more commonly referred to as chicken-pox.
13. Subacute sclerosing panencephalitis is a rare complication of measles; it is a progressive, lethal neu-rological disease.

True or False

1. False
2. True F,,
3. True
4. True
5. True

Fill in the Blank

1. subacute sclerosing panencephalitis
2. CD8+ T cells
3. Koplik's spots
4. gamma globulin
5. parotid

Multiple Choice

1. e A,
2. b c,
3. a .
4. b c,

Critical Thinking Exercise

1. Tom's reference to danger associated with measles and pregnancy is congenital rubella syndrome. If rubella is acquired during the first trimester, it can be spread via the placenta to the fetus with birth defects like cardiac anomalies, deafness, and mental retardation possible.
2. There are two types of measles: red measles or rubeola and German measles or rubella. They are caused by two different viruses. Rubella is typically a mild disease characterized by the develop-ment of a discrete pink maculopapular rash appearing on the face and spreading peripherally to the extremities. Rubeola is characterized by runny nose, fever, cough, sneezing, and Koplick's spots on the mouth epithelium.
3. Presence of IgM is diagnostic for a recent infection of red measles virus after a presumptive diag-nosis based on clinical symptoms. ELISAs are available for detection of anti-measles IgM or anti-measles IgG. Serological tests to detect the presence of antibodies to the E1, E2, or the nucleocapsid protein C are available for rubella virus. Attenuvax is a vaccine available for red measles virus, and Meruvax II is available for vaccination against rubella.

Case Study

1. Presumptive diagnosis is mumps. Cause is the mumps virus, which is a member of the *Paramyx-oviridae*, and spread is via the upper respiratory route with primary viral replication in mucosal ep-ithelium and lymphocytes in that region.

2. The incubation period for mumps is two to three weeks with swelling of the parotids generally apparent for 7 to 10 days. Humoral and cellular immune components participate in immunological responses to all viral infections. When virus is outside the cells, humoral immunity is activated; cellular immunity becomes the key player when the virus is inside the cell. Mucosal immunity occurs in the lamina propria, and dimeric IgA antibodies are secreted from plasma cells that activate classical complement pathway and prevents the virus from absorbing to the mucosal epithelium and lymphocytes.
3. Complications of mumps include meningitis, pancreatitis, and neurosensory deafness. Mumps encephalitis occurs in about 1% of infections, but for the 14-year-old boy a likelihood of substantial swelling of the testicles (since he is post pubertal) with sterility is a rarity but not unknown as a complication.

CHAPTER 21

Matching

1. q
2. j
3. u
4. f
5. c
6. m
7. o
8. a
9. d
10. s
11. r
12. g
13. p
14. h
15. l
16. i
17. t
18. k
19. b
20. n
21. e

Definitions

1. Acute phase refers to the period of the disease process in which the virus is fully active.
2. Adenoids are lymphatic tissues in the recess of the nasopharynx.
3. Adenovirus is a common pathogen of the *Adenoviridae* family; a naked DNA virus.
4. An adjuvant is a substance added to a vaccine to enhance the immune response so a higher antibody titer is achieved.
5. Antigenic drift refers to minor mutations in HA and NA.
6. Antigenic shift refers to major changes in HA and NA.

7. Cytomegalovirus (CMV) is a virus that is a member of the *Herpesviridae* family consisting of double-stranded DNA that is prevalent in the general population and is usually asymptomatic except in the immunosuppressed and neonates.
8. Asymptomatic refers to being free of signs and symptoms of disease or infection.
9. Epstein Barr virus (EBV) is a virus that is a member of the *Herpesviridae* family consisting of double-stranded DNA, which causes infectious mononucleosis.
10. The convalescent phase refers to the period of a disease in which the virus is diminishing.
11. Immunocompetent refers to being able to fight off disease and infection.
12. Infectious mononucleosis refers to an infectious disease infecting the lymphoid tissues caused by infection with the Epstein-Barr virus.
13. Poliovirus is a virus that is a member of the *Picornaviridae* family consisting of small naked virions with an RNA genome enclosed within an icosahedral capsid.

True or False

1. False
2. True
3. True
4. True
5. True

Fill in the Blank

1. adenoids
2. endocytosis
3. vector
4. CMV
5. CytoGam

Multiple Choice

1. c
2. e
3. b
4. a

Critical Thinking Exercise

1. Epstein Barr virus (EBV) causes infectious mononucleosis (IM). The virus is infectious meaning it will cause infection given the right circumstances (like repeated contact with an infected individual generally requiring salivary contact), but it is not so contagious given its typical mode of transmission. So unless intimate contact is in the near future with the student sitting next to you, the opportunity for transmission is very remote.
2. The virus is transmitted via salivary contact generally. The primary cell target for EBV infection is the B cell. Investigators, Epstein and Barr, first identified the virus in tumors from Ugandan children. EBV infection is associated with Burkitt's lymphoma (B cell malignancy) and a tumor of the nasal passages (nasopharyngeal carcinoma).
3. Acute clinical disease may manifest as sore throat, extreme fatigue, and malaise. EBV acts like a commensal organism in equilibrium with the host, the virus remaining dormant in cells for life. EBV hinders the hydrolysis of viral peptides by the proteasome, so the communication process by which the immune system identifies infected cells has been disrupted. Also, EBV inhibits signals that would normally induce the infected cell to commit cell suicide (apoptosis) ensuring the viral factory will

not be destroyed. EBV infected individuals may have antibodies to a red blood cell antigen (gly-cophorin). These anti-red blood cell antibodies can result in anemia as a result of complement activation on the red blood cell.

4. Heterophile antibodies are other antibodies produced during EBV induced infectious mononucleosis, but are cross-reactive with antigen in another species. They are not specific to EBV. Diagnosis of IM was routinely based on the detection of the heterophile antibodies that would agglutinate horse, sheep, and bovine erythrocytes. While there are vaccines available for EBV, the live attenuated vaccines (which are most effective) have problems since the virus is associated with some forms of cancer. Recombinant EBV vaccines have been tested in clinical trials, however.

5. Diagnosis of IM was based on assays measuring heterophile antibodies for many years because they can be detected in 80 to 90% of individuals infected with EBV. The classic test was the Paul-Bunnell Davidsohn Differential Test. More recently serological tests based on detection of antibodies specific for EBV have become commercially available.

CHAPTER 22

Matching

1. h
2. p
3. a
4. l
5. j
6. c
7. e
8. n
9. f
10. b
11. i
12. d
13. o
14. m
15. g
16. k

Definitions

1. Acid citrate dextrose is an anticoagulant.
2. Acquired immunodeficiency syndrome is the final stage of infection with HIV characterized by the complete breakdown of the immune system.
3. Amplicor HIV monitor test is an assay for measurement of HIV-1 in plasma.
4. Antibody capture is the binding of the patient's antibodies to Fc regions.
5. The human immunodeficiency virus is the causative agent for AIDS; it is a member of the *Retroviridae* family of viruses.
6. Human T cell leukemia viruses are also members of the *Retroviridae*; there are three identified in humans; HTVL-1 is associated with adult T cell leukemia (ATL).
7. Hypergammaglobulinemia refers to an increased level of circulating antibodies.
8. Langerhans cells refer to alpha, beta, and delta cells in the pancreas responsible for the production of insulin, secretion of glucagon, and the inhibition of the secretion of growth hormone.

9. Modified vaccinia ankara strain refers to a virus in which some viral genes have been excised and HIV genes have been inserted.
10. Prime-boost refers to a DNA vaccine injected at a later time with a recombinant protein.
11. A provirus is integrated viral RNA; proviral DNA.
12. Retroviruses are enveloped single-stranded RNA viruses whose RNA genome is converted into double-stranded DNA following host cell entry.
13. Tropical spastic paraparesis is a chronic degenerative neurological disease; HTVL-1 associated myelopathy (HAM).

True or False

1. True
2. True
3. False
4. True
5. True

Fill in the Blank

1. Retroviruses
2. Integrase, reverse transcriptase, and viral protease
3. virions
4. provirus
5. AIDS

Multiple Choice

1. e
2. d
3. b
4. a

Critical Thinking Exercise

1. Seroconversion is B cell activation and differentiation to antibody secreting cells (resulting in detectable anti-HIV antibodies) and is usually apparent within one month but may not be detectable for three to six months following infection. Studies of people repeatedly exposed to HIV in high-risk situations who do not develop circulating anti-HIV antibodies (seroconvert) have been the subject of many investigations. Maybe the immune system under certain circumstances may eliminate the virus, or individuals with homozygous deletion or some sort of genetic modification of the co-receptor CCR5 make up a large percent of the individuals resistant to HIV infection. Some infected are also slow progressors to AIDS.
2. Circumcision would remove the Langerhans cells isolated from male foreskin epithelia, which are infected first and carry the infection (present antigen) into the nearest lymph node and a CD4+ T cell. Some controversial research has demonstrated that male circumcision might slow the advance of AIDS throughout Africa.
3. Opportunistic infections/malignancies, prevalent due to significant loss of CD4+ T cells, include *Candida*, Cytomegalovirus, lymphoma, Kaposi's sarcoma, Herpes simplex virus, *Mycobacterium tuberculosis*, and *Pneumocystis carinii*.
4. Intradermal or subcutaneous injections of recombinant proteins have been the focus of many trials for the more than 30 candidate HIV vaccines. HIV gp120 recombinant protein is the antigen used in the vaccine marketed as AIDSVAX. Live attenuated viruses carry the risk of reversion to the wild

type such as has happened with poliovirus. Molecular biology techniques have also been used in working on a vaccine for HIV using plasmid DNA as a vaccine, although the magnitude of responses has not been sufficiently high to ensure protection. A strategy using protein injections or genetically altered viruses along with the DNA vaccine is called a prime-boost approach.

5. Serological tests that measure anti-HIV antibodies are the basis for HIV screening. Various enzyme immunoassays are available, but the ELISA is the most commonly used platform. Most of the antibody tests use one of the following three approaches: indirect enzyme immunoassay, double antigen sandwich technique, or antibody or antigen capture techniques. Serum samples can be obtained safely through OraSure.

CHAPTER 23

Matching

1. g
2. u
3. n
4. a
5. q
6. j
7. s
8. o
9. l
10. t
11. c
12. e
13. i
14. p
15. h
16. r
17. b
18. m
19. k
20. d
21. f

Definitions

1. Aflatoxin is a toxin made when *Aspergillus* grows on peanuts, wheat, or rice.
2. Asexual means without male or female reproductive organs.
3. Aspergillosis refers to an invasive pulmonary infection caused by *Aspergillus*.
4. *Aspergillus* spores are airborne particles from *Aspergillus spp*.
5. *Candida albicans* is an infectious disease-causing fungus.
6. *Cryptococcus neoformans* is an encapsulated yeast-like fungus found in pigeon roosts and in soil containing pigeon or chicken droppings.
7. Mucocutaneous candidiasis refers to a skin infection with *C. albicans*.
8. Thrush refers to *Candida* infection presenting as white, cheesy plaque on mucosae.
9. Vaginal candidiasis refers to a *Candida* infection with thick yellow or milky discharge.
10. Opportunistic refers to fungi causing disease in immunocompromised hosts.

11. Normal flora are microorganisms present naturally in the environment.
12. Nitric oxide is produced when inducible nitric oxide synthase is activated, and it is one of three types of cytotoxic molecules in the macrophage that enable it to destroy organisms present in the phagocytic vacuole.
13. The murex cryptococcal test is a rapid, point-of-care test that detects cryptococcal polysaccharides.

True or False

1. True
2. True
3. True
4. False
5. True

Fill in the Blank

1. Aspergillosis
2. opportunistic
3. aflatoxin
4. immunocompetent
5. Mycetomas (fungal balls)

Multiple Choice

1. a
2. b
3. a
4. d

Critical Thinking Exercise

1. When the immune system is disrupted, particularly cellular immunity, *Candida albicans* can cause chronic infection. Patients with inserted lines (urinary tract catheters for example) are also at risk for infection because *Candida* adheres to the plastic material used in their construction. Past history and the immunosuppression via prolonged antibiotic therapy are complicating factors in Theresa's medical history, too. Since *Candida* is part of the natural flora, they compete with resident bacteria for an ecological niche in mucus membranes. Theresa's prolonged antibiotic therapy allowed *Candida* to out-compete normal resident bacteria and dominate. If the fungi convert to the pseudohyphal form, they may disseminate to deeper tissues especially in light of Theresa's problem with decubitus ulcers (bed sores) where areas of the epidermis are absent as the initial immune protection.
2. Diseases range from superficial skin and mucous infections (mucocutaneous candidiasis) to disseminated systemic infection of many organs. Pseudohyphae secrete enzymes facilitating tissue invasion. Acute cutaneous candidiasis may occur in individuals who are not severely immunocompromised. *Candida* is controlled by the immune system and environmental factors such as pH.
3. Candida exists primarily in a yeast form with blastoconidia extending out from the cell as asexual reproduction. Pseudohyphae form when these buds remain attached to the main body. Under some circumstances, true hyphae may form. *Candida* is considered dimorphic. Pseudohyphae bind to a number of tissues (for example, collagen).
4. In one study based on a murine model, immunization using mannan extracts encapsulated in liposomes resulted in generation of protective antibodies. Subsequent challenge with *C. albicans* afforded protection against disseminated disease.

5. Diagnosis of *C. albicans* is based on identification of the organism in culture or direct microscopy with slides from swab specimens. Diagnosis of invasive candidiasis is made using PCR along with biotinylated primers for easy detection.

CHAPTER 24

Matching

1. m
2. q
3. n
4. a
5. u
6. k
7. d
8. b
9. s
10. f
11. h
12. p
13. c
14. t
15. g
16. l
17. e
18. o
19. j
20. i
21. r

Definitions

1. Ameba refers to a small unicellular organism moving by pseudopodia.
2. Amebic colitis is a disease of the large intestine caused by *Entamoeba histolytica*.
3. Bradyzoites are the dormant form of *Toxoplasma gondii* occupying cysts in infected tissues.
4. Congenital toxoplasmosis is a severe form of toxoplasmosis contracted by pregnant women.
5. The definitive host refers to the organism in which larvae develop into adult worms.
6. Echinococcosis is a larval tapeworm infection caused by ingestion of egg-contaminated food.
7. Erythrocytes are red blood cells.
8. Hepatocytes are liver parenchyma cells.
9. Hydatid cysts are tissue growths resulting from parasitic worm infection.
10. An intermediate host is one in which eggs develop into larvae but do not mature into adult worms.
11. Merozoite microgametocytes are male merozoites that merge with megagametocytes to produce zygotes in *Plasmodium spp.*
12. Protoscoleces are immature tapeworm heads.
13. A zygote refers to the fertilized cell resulting from the merging of a microgametocyte with a megagametocyte in *Plasmodium spp.*

True or False

1. False
2. True
3. False
4. True
5. False

Fill in the Blank

1. obligate parasites
2. pseudopodia
3. *Acanthamoeba spp.* and *Naegleria fowleri*
4. granulomas
5. Amebic keratitis

Multiple Choice

1. e
2. a
3. b
4. d

Critical Thinking Exercise

1. The definitive host for *Plasmodium spp.* is the *Anopheles* mosquito because reproduction occurs in the mosquito, but humans are intermediate hosts. Having two different hosts may benefit *Plasmodium* by extending its range or protecting it when one of the hosts is removed by some circumstance. *Plasmodium* may be controlled by controlling mosquitoes.
2. Patients with sickle cell anemia (inherited trait affecting hemoglobin molecule) infected with *Plasmodium spp.* may not develop malaria because the parasite cannot survive in red blood cells that are sickle shaped. It is thought the sickle cell anemia trait evolved under malarial conditions.
3. The generalized life cycle involves liver parenchyma cells (hepatocytes) and the red blood cell (erythrocytes). The life cycle is complex but understanding of the cycle is essential before considering immunology of infection or problems associated with vaccine development. Sporozoites (motile infective form) enter the blood stream as a result of a mosquito "bite," and travel to the liver where they infect the hepatocytes. Schizonts (multinucleated form) develop and their nuclei are encapsulated to form merozoites. Merozoites released from the liver bind to specific receptors and enter the red blood cell. Inside the erythrocyte the malarial parasite endocytoses much of the hemoglobin differentiating into a trophozoite (ring form). Trophozoites undergo a development cycle in the red blood cell like the sporozoites do in the liver, and schizonts form and nuclei encapsulate to form merozoites again. A small number of released merozoites become either microgametocytes (males) or megagametocytes (females) that are gamete forms. These gamete forms do not develop into zygotes unless the definitive host (the mosquito) ingests them in a blood meal. Antigenic epitopes differ on the two parasitic forms (sporozoite and merozoite), so immunity generated against one does not affect the other. Individuals develop antibodies to the antigens present on the two parasitic forms, so individuals continue to have low level parasitemia with minimal symptomology.
4. Malarial pigment is produced by the incomplete metabolism of hemoglobin by the merozoites. Clinical manifestations of infection with *Plasmodium spp.* are cyclic fever (action of macrophage-derived cytokines on brain tissues correlated with cyclic lysis of red blood cells), malaise, myalgia, anemia, and headache. Some acquired immunity is presumed in areas where malaria is endemic because the incidence and severity decrease with age.

5. Because the malarial parasite has both intracellular and extracellular stages, the development of an effective vaccine is challenging. Vaccine design, therefore, must be based on consideration of the complex life cycle and the requirements for both humoral and cellular immunity.
6. Definitive diagnosis of malaria requires direct observation in stained (Giemsa) blood smears. Commercially available tests detect anti-malarial antibodies, malarial antigens (HRP-2), or malarial enzymes (parasitic lactate dehydrogenase).

CHAPTER 25

Matching

1. u
2. e
3. m
4. h
5. p
6. c
7. r
8. t
9. a
10. o
11. f
12. q
13. b
14. g
15. s
16. k
17. n
18. i
19. l
20. d
21. j

Definitions

1. Anti-double-stranded DNA refers to an autoantibody present in systemic lupus erythematosus.
2. Autoantibody is an antibody specific for self protein.
3. The butterfly rash is a characteristic mark on the face as a result of systemic lupus erythematosus.
4. Diabetes mellitus is a chronic autoimmune disease resulting from a disorder of glucose metabolism in which too little insulin is produced.
5. Glutamic acid decarboxylase is an autoantibody to the beta islet cell enzyme.
6. Graves' disease is an autoimmune disease in which autoantibodies stimulate the thyroid gland.
7. Hashimoto's thyroiditis is an autoimmune disease resulting in hypothyroidism.
8. Insulin is a hormone secreted by the pancreas essential to cellular use of glucose to produce energy.
9. Intrinsic factor is a protein necessary for the transport of vitamin B12 from the intestine to the blood.
10. Parietal cells are the cells lining the gastrointestinal tract.
11. Pernicious anemia is a condition manifesting as severe chronic gastritis.
12. Rheumatoid arthritis is a chronic systemic inflammatory disorder with unknown etiology.
13. Synovium refers to fluid in the joints.

True or False

1. True
2. False
3. False
4. True
5. True

Fill in the Blank

1. rate nephelometry
2. SLE
3. genetic
4. butterfly rash
5. double-stranded DNA

Multiple Choice

1. b
2. e
3. c
4. e

Critical Thinking/Case Study Exercise

1. Pernicious anemia. Severe chronic gastritis is connected to pernicious anemia because the breakdown in self-tolerance creates antibodies that attack proteins in the gastric mucosa (parietal cells).
2. Underlying cause of pernicious anemia is malabsorption of vitamin B12 because the intrinsic factor (a protein) required for transport of vitamin B12 from intestine to the blood is lacking. Clinical scenarios leading to pernicious anemia include gastrectomy, antibody-mediated destruction of parietal cells that produce intrinsic factor, or binding of antibodies to intrinsic factors. (B12 is requisite for erythropoiesis.)
3. Parietal cells produce intrinsic factor that is necessary for the absorption of vitamin B12 from intestine to blood. Absorption only occurs when vitamin B12 combines with the protein, intrinsic factor, made by parietal cells of the stomach mucosa. Tests to determine whether the vitamin B12 deficiency is due to impaired absorption or to dietary deficiency include the Schilling test. Serological tests determine the presence of antibodies to intrinsic factor. Indirect immunofluorescent antibody technique is used to detect anti-parietal cell antibodies.

CHAPTER 26

Matching

1. h
2. t
3. m
4. a
5. o
6. r
7. d

8. i
9. e
10. s
11. f
12. q
13. b
14. l
15. j
16. n
17. k
18. c
19. p
20. g

Definitions

1. Acute leukemia refers to excessive proliferation of a developing white blood cell that has failed to mature.
2. Acute lymphoblastic leukemia is a more common form of the disease that may have a genetic component.
3. Acute myelogenous leukemia is characterized by sudden onset of the disease with a short life expectancy without treatment.
4. Alpha-fetoprotein is a tumor associated oncofetal antigen secreted normally during fetal development.
5. Bence Jones proteins are monoclonal proteins detected in urine.
6. Beta-human chorionic gonadotrophin is a tumor associated oncofetal antigen; the beta chain of a dimeric oncofetal protein associated with pregnancy and some forms of cancer.
7. Burkitt's lymphoma is associated with Epstein Barr virus and the viral genome is present in all tumor cells in endemic areas.
8. Carcinoembryonic antigen is a tumor associated oncofetal antigen; a membrane protein found in serum.
9. Chronic leukemia is the form of the disease in which the malignant cell is a mature white blood cell.
10. Tumor specific antigens are antigens unique to the tumor.
11. Determinant selection refers to the absence of the interaction of MHC molecules with antigenic peptides to form complexes.
12. Receptor idiotype refers to receptors whose variable regions are specific to a particular clone.
13. Philadelphia chromosome refers to a genetically altered chromosome 22.

True or False

1. True
2. False
3. False
4. True
5. True

Fill in the Blank

1. galactin 9
2. receptor idiotype
3. oncofetal antigens

4. macrophages
5. costimulatory

Multiple Choice

1. a
2. d
3. a
4. c

Critical Thinking/Case Study Exercise

1. Nursing and immunology classes "share" the following pathologies concerning hemopoiesis and myeloid and lymphoid stem cells: acute leukemias (lymphoblastic, B cell, T cell, myelogenous), chronic leukemias (lymphocytic, B cell, T cell, myelogenous), lymphomas (Hodgkin's, non-Hodgkin's, B cell, T cell), and plasma cell dyscrasia.

2. Immunophenotyping analysis is based on targeting of cell markers with fluorescently labeled antibody detected by flow cytometry. Malignant cells in acute myelogenous leukemia carry the CD33 and CD13 markers, while malignant B cell blasts, characteristic of acute lymphoblastic leukemia, express CD19 and CD10 cell surface markers. Markers present on malignant T cell blasts are CD2, CD5, and CD7 with cytoplasmic CD3. Chronic myelogenous leukemia is characterized by a chromosome abnormality known as the Philadelphia chromosome, which is a genetically altered chromosome 22. Segments of chromosomes 9 and 22 are switched. The new sequence on chromosome 22 encodes a protein, BCR-ABL (a tyrosine kinase).

3. Myeloid (myelogenous) neoplasms occur in myeloid cell lineages, whereas lymphoid (lymphocytic) neoplasms occur in lymphoid cell lineages. Acute refers to excessive proliferation of immature forms, whereas chronic refers to excessive proliferation of mature forms of the cell line in question. Lymphomas include Hodgkin's (uncommon disorder characterized by Reed-Sternberg cells that are distinctive giant cells) or non-Hodgkin's (heterogeneous group of lymphoid malignancies whose incidence increases with age and immunosuppression). Mechanisms proposed by which tumors may evade the immune system fall into the three following categories: tumor antigen related (absence of antigen specific receptor or hole in the repertoire phenomenon), class I MHC related (absence of an appropriate MHC allele), or T cell related (complexity of costimulatory molecules).

CHAPTER 27

Matching

1. m
2. s
3. k
4. p
5. i
6. r
7. a
8. o
9. c
10. q
11. g
12. b

13. e
14. h
15. n
16. d
17. j
18. l
19. f

Definitions

1. Bruton's agammaglobulinemia refers to an immunodeficiency disorder linked to the X chromosome.
2. CD55 refers to a regulatory complement protein; also known as decay accelerating factor.
3. Chediak Higashi syndrome is a multi-system immunodeficiency disorder in which patients are susceptible to a variety of pathogens.
4. DiGeorge's syndrome is a primary immunodeficiency disorder associated with T cell immunity.
5. Giant cytoplasmic granules are a characteristic of Chediak Higashi syndrome resulting from uncontrolled fusion of granules.
6. Hereditary angioneurotic edema is a life-threatening edema in which there is swelling of the face, larynx, and gastrointestinal tract.
7. Immunoglobulin deficiency with increased IgM refers to a primary immunodeficiency disorder in which there is an increased level of serum IgM but a decrease in IgG, IgA, and IgE.
8. Leukocyte adhesion deficiency (LAD) is a disorder in which phagocytes lack the cell surface molecules through which they would normally adhere to other leukocytes.
9. Malnutrition is a lack of essential substances in one's diet.
10. Paroxysmal nocturnal hemoglobinuria is a disorder in which membrane attack complexes form on red blood cells resulting in lysis.
11. SCID is an immunodeficiency that affects both T cells and B cells.
12. Therapeutic gamma globulin is an injection of gamma globulin from donor serum.
13. Selective IgA deficiency is the most common immunodeficiency disorder exhibited by a diminished level of serum IgA; B cells do not differentiate to IgA.

True or False

1. True
2. False
3. False
4. False
5. True

Fill in the Blank

1. recurrent sinopulmonary infection
2. DiGeorge's syndrome
3. thymus
4. adenosine deaminase
5. Wiskott Aldrich syndrome

Multiple Choice

1. a
2. a
3. d
4. c

Critical Thinking Exercise

1. Bruton's agammaglobulinemia (XLA) is an immunodeficiency disorder linked to the X chromosome. It is not the most common immunodeficiency disorder; that is selective IgA deficiency.
2. XLA is apparent at around 6 to 9 months of age because that time corresponds to when most of the mother's antibodies crossing the placenta have been degraded. Viral infections are not affected since T cell immunity is intact, but bacterial infections of the upper respiratory tract are common presentations. Treatment is intravenous therapeutic gamma globulin (antibody) therapy pooled from donor sera following screening for hepatitis and immunodeficiency virus.
3. In Bruton's agammaglobulinemia (XLA), serum levels of IgA and IgM are undetectable, and IgG is present at very low levels. XLA is a defect in a gene coding for a signaling tyrosine kinase. Without the signaling event the pre-B cells do not develop and mature into B cells with the subsequent gross deficiency of mature B cells and immunoglobulins.

CHAPTER 28

Matching

1. f
2. e
3. m
4. q
5. b
6. n
7. a
8. j
9. o
10. g
11. l
12. p
13. h
14. r
15. d
16. i
17. c
18. k

Definitions

1. Hypersensitivity reactions are immunological responses not controlled by normal regulatory mechanisms.
2. Type I hypersensitivity reactions are immediate hypersensitivity or IgE-mediated reactions like allergies, rhinitis, and anaphylaxis.
3. Type II hypersensitivity reactions are those in which production of IgG and IgM antibodies target cell surface antigens causing pathologies like hemolytic disease of the newborn, autoimmune disorders, drug-induced reactions, and transfusion reactions.
4. Type III hypersensitivity reactions are those in which IgG and IgM antibodies target soluble antigens and large immune complexes form as in SLE, post streptococcal glomerulonephritis, serum sickness, and farmer's lung.

5. Type IV hypersensitivity reactions are cell mediated. The effector phase is referred to as delayed type hypersensitivity (DTH) responses, and clinical examples would include chronic infection with *Mycobacterium tuberculosis* and poison ivy dermatitis.
6. Anaphylaxis is a potentially fatal immediate hypersensitivity response with cardiac and respiratory symptoms.
7. Desensitization refers to treatments called allergy shots in which the rationale for the treatment is that the injection of antigen, in small doses, will trigger isotype switching of newly activated B cell clones from IgM to IgG.
8. Hemolytic disease of the newborn occurs when a mother, whose red blood cells do not express the Rh antigen (Rh negative), is carrying a fetus that is Rh positive. If maternal anti-Rh IgG antibodies cross the placenta and bind to antigen on fetal red blood cells, the red blood cells are destroyed leading to anemia in the fetus.
9. Haptens are too small to trigger an immune response on their own, but they function as epitopes attached to a larger molecule, referred to as a carrier.
10. Goodpasture's syndrome occurs when antibodies bind to antigens present on kidney and lung membranes causing cell damage.
11. Myasthenia gravis is an autoimmune disease in which autoantibodies bind to epitopes on acetylcholine receptors in the motor-end plate of the neuromuscular junction, thereby blocking acetylcholine-mediated neuromuscular transmission.
12. Isohemagglutinins are natural IgM antibodies that are generated without exposure to the antigens "A" or "B" but rather to exposure to bacterial antigens in the gut that are cross-reactive with the antigens present on the red blood cells.

True or False

1. False
2. True
3. False
4. False
5. True

Fill in the Blank

1. Basophils
2. Mast cells
3. Anaphylaxis
4. epinephrine
5. histamine

Multiple Choice

1. e
2. b
3. c
4. c

Critical Thinking Exercise

1. Gell and Coombs system, or a modified version of this system, classifies all hypersensitivity reactions as Type I (immediate hypersensitivity), Type II (antibody mediated), Type III (immune complex mediated), and Type IV (T cell mediated).

2. Allergies and anaphylaxis fit into Type I hypersensitivity reactions, while contact dermatitis fits under the Type IV hypersensitivity reaction (variant delayed type response). Sensitization phase refers to the initial immunological response following exposure to an antigen, while the effector phase refers to subsequent immunological responses to that antigen and clinical manifestations.

3. Atopic individuals develop allergies, and atopy refers to IgE-mediated allergic reactions. Atopic individuals have a predominance of CD4+ cells that secrete Type 2 cytokines, which determine the isotype switching to IgE. (Cytokines are a contributing factor in the microenvironment determining the particular isotype to which switching will occur.) Prophylactic treatment of atopic individuals includes anti-histamine drugs preventing histamine, which is released by degranulation of basophils and mast cells, from binding to histamine receptors. Stabilizers of the mast cell/basophil membrane like sodium cromoglycate are available, but for those experiencing anaphylaxis, epinephrine is injected for immediate action. Transplants are Type II, and DTH response is Type IV. Persistent infections are Type III in general although a chronic DTH or Type IV response is associated with individuals infected with *Mycobacterium tuberculosis*.